Psychiatric Nursing Research

WILEY SERIES ON
DEVELOPMENTS IN NURSING RESEARCH

Series Editor

Jenifer Wilson-Barnett
Reader in Nursing Studies, King's College, University of London

Volume 1
Recovery from Illness
JENIFER WILSON-BARNETT AND MORVA FORDHAM

Volume 2
Nursing Research: Ten Studies in Patient Care
Edited by
JENIFER WILSON-BARNETT

Volume 3
Psychiatric Nursing Research
Edited by
JULIA BROOKING
Lecturer in Nursing Studies, King's College, University of London

Volume 4
Research in Preventive Community Nursing Care   (in press)
Edited by
ALISON WHILE
Department of Nursing Studies, King's College, University of London

Volume 5
Research in Geriatric Nursing   (in preparation)
Edited by
PAULINE FIELDING
Director of Clinical Nursing Research, The Middlesex Hospital, London

WILEY SERIES ON
DEVELOPMENTS IN NURSING RESEARCH
VOLUME 3

Psychiatric Nursing Research

edited by

JULIA BROOKING
Lecturer in Nursing Studies
King's College
University of London, UK

A Wiley Medical Publication

JOHN WILEY & SONS
Chichester · New York · Brisbane · Toronto · Singapore

Library of Congress Cataloging in Publication Data:

Main entry under title:
Psychiatric nursing research.

  (Wiley series on developments in nursing research; v.3)
(A Wiley medical publication)
  Includes bibliographies and index.
  1. Psychiatric nursing.   2. Psychiatric nursing — Research.
I. Brooking, Julia.   II. Series.
III. Series: A Wiley medical publication.
[DNLM: 1. Psychiatric Nursing.   2. Research.
W1 WI53LF v.3 / WY 160 P97405]
  RC440.P77 1986   610.73'68'072   85-20402

ISBN 0 471 90907 6 (pbk.)

British Library Cataloguing in Publication Data:

Psychiatric nursing research. — (Wiley series on
  developments in nursing research; 3) — (A Wiley
  medical publication)
  1. Psychiatric nursing
  I. Brooking, Julia   II. Series
  610.73'68   RC440

ISBN 0 471 90907 6

Phototypeset by Dobbie Typesetting Service, Plymouth, Devon
Printed and bound in Great Britain

List of Contributors

ANNIE ALTSCHUL, CBE, BA, MSc, SRN, RMN, RNT, FRCN   Emeritus Professor of Nursing Studies, University of Edinburgh

CHARLES BROOKER, BA, RMN, JBCNS Course 650   Senior Nurse (Research and Planning), Mental Health Unit, Bloomsbury Health Authority, London

JULIA BROOKING, BSc, SRN, RMN, DipN, Cert Ed, RNT   Lecturer in Nursing Studies, University of London, King's College

MARTIN BROWN, RMN, RCNT, JBCNS Course 650   Assistant Nurse Adviser, Society of Psychiatric and Mental Handicap Nursing, Royal College of Nursing of the United Kingdom

BRYN DAVIS, BSc, PhD, SRN, RMN, RNT   Principal Lecturer, Department of Community Studies, Brighton Polytechnic

NANCY FARLEY, BA, SRN, RMN, SCM, Certificate in Behavioural Psychotherapy   Director of Nursing, Hayes Grove Priory Hospital, Kent

VERONA GORDON, RN, BSN, MS, PhD   Professor, School of Nursing, University of Minnesota, USA

KEVIN GOURNAY, MPhil, RMN, RNMH, JBCNS Course 650   Senior Nurse/ Behaviour Therapist, Barnet General Hospital, Hertfordshire, and University of Leicester, Psychology Department

R. GLYN JONES, BSc, RMN   Senior Nurse (Research) Murray Royal Hospital, Perth, Scotland

EIMEAR MUIR-COCHRANE, BSc, SRN   Psychiatric Student Nurse, The Bethlem Royal and Maudsley Hospitals, London

MARION TALMADGE REED, RN, BSN, MN, RMN, RGN   Manager, Broadfields Day Centre, Barnet, Hertfordshire and Psychiatric Clinical Nurse Specialist, USA

FRED ROACH, BA, MSc, RMN, CertEd, RNT   Lecturer, Institute of Advanced
    Nursing Education, Royal College of Nursing of the United Kingdom
DAVID SKIDMORE, MSc, RMN, RCNT, Teacher's Certificate   Senior Lecturer in
    Nursing, Manchester Polytechnic
JOSEPHINE TISSIER, BSc, SRN   Staff Nurse, St. George's Hospital, London
EDWARD WHITE, MSc, RMN, Diploma in Community Psychiatric Nursing   Senior
    Nurse (Health Care Research) Maidstone Health Authority, Kent and
    Honorary Research Fellow, Health Services Research Unit, University
    of Kent at Canterbury

Contents

Series Preface

Developments in Nursing Research

Nursing science is derived from an integration of knowledge in other disciplines and from original nursing research studies. As more relevant research is completed key areas are developing, benefiting from different approaches in various patient care settings. The purpose of this series is to publish literature reviews and original material in such areas to promote nursing progress and knowledge.

Foreword

All professions are in quest of theory and hope to find it emerging from research. The nursing profession has not yet moved far in this quest, least of all in the psychiatric part of it. It has made some progress, however, in that area of the research enterprise which is meant to benefit the consumers. Such research is encouraged by Government since it is expected to lead to improved services and greater cost effectiveness. If such research is to result in change of practice it is necessary that new studies should follow from the conclusions of previous research and that each study should generate ideas from which inspiration for new researchers will derive. This book represents an attempt to help British nurses along this path. Psychiatric nurses have not in the past been well served. From this collection of papers they will get an overview of the relevant research territory and a glimpse of the way ahead.

The Editor's introductory remarks and Bryn Davis' review accurately reflect the present state of ignorance in the field and point the way psychiatric nurses might contribute to fill the void.

The book contains reports of ten small studies and an account of eight students' projects. All of these stand alone, their authors crying out for support or refutation from others.

The consumers who are least well served are patients in mental hospitals. Only two of the students' projects address themselves to their cause. Those whose care takes place in the community fare slightly better and a group of 'not-yet patients', that is of self-referred depressed women, has been the subject of a well controlled study of nursing effectiveness. Nurses who work in specialist areas, such as behaviour modification and in the community, have studied their clients a little more persistently.

The consumers who will derive most benefit from this book are nurses—not patients. Student nurses, nurse-educators and nurse-managers will learn much from the questions posed by the researchers and from the discussion of their findings. Six of the papers and six of the students' projects deal with various aspects of 'when, how and where' to deploy nurses with diverse levels of skill, knowledge and experience.

The immediate benefit will accrue to researchers. Each and every paper poses questions about methodology. Each provides hypotheses for future research.

In my opinion too many express doubt about the validity of their research. Too many point to the limitation of small samples and warn about generalizing. Why should nurses have so many scruples about sample size? Doctors are quite happy to research and report research from the very limited case material available to them. The edifice of psychoanalysis rests on very few cases. Knowledge builds up gradually, by piecing together findings from little studies, replicated and elaborated on later. It is proper for students of research to disarm their examiners by pointing out limitations but not for serious researchers to be paralysed by diffidence.

I believe that this book will have considerable impetus on psychiatric nurses and will soon have to be followed by a new report of the research it has helped to inspire.

Annie Altschul

Introduction

JULIA BROOKING

For a long time psychiatric nursing has drawn on research carried out by other disciplines, but research by psychiatric nurses about psychiatric nursing is of relatively recent origin. This is the first British collection of psychiatric nursing studies brought together in a single volume. It represents a variety of research approaches, using different methods and investigating a range of problems.

The main aim of this volume is to provide an overview of the 'state of the art' of psychiatric nursing research. Most of the contributors are British and the two American researchers have recently worked in Britain. Given the newness of psychiatric nursing as an academic discipline and the paucity of research, it is inevitable that all the studies in this book can be criticized. In most cases the authors are very aware of the limitations and methodological flaws in their work and would welcome critical comments from readers. This book is probably a fairly accurate reflection of the range and variety of psychiatric nursing research studies in the mid 1980s.

The second aim is to give readers some indicators for practice and for further research. There is always a danger in trying to make generalizations from small unrepresentative studies, but nevertheless these chapters do provide many useful pointers by identifying deficient practices, showing gaps in service provision, and identifying areas for clinical, educational, and research developments.

This is the first book of its type. All the chapters are written by psychiatric nurses and concern some aspect of psychiatric nursing practice or education. It is doubtful whether such a collection could have been compiled in Britain ten or fifteen years ago. Even today it was difficult to find sufficient recently completed studies for this volume. The development of psychiatric nursing research has lagged behind nursing research generally, for reasons partly associated with the lack of adequate educational opportunities available for psychiatric nurses (Brooking, 1984). For example, of the twenty or more undergraduate degrees in or with nursing offered at British universities and polytechnics, only three combine with registration in psychiatric nursing as opposed to general nursing. This is important because it is at degree level study that competence to carry out research is likely to be first developed. Most of the contributors to this book have had to take time out from their chosen profession to read for degrees in other disciplines, such as psychology and sociology.

The range of topics examined in these chapters is of interest. Recent major studies have tended to concern specialized rather than general roles, e.g. evaluation of community psychiatric nursing (Paykel and Griffiths, 1983) and nurse behaviour therapy (Marks *et al.*, 1977). When planning this book it became obvious that this trend has continued. It was relatively easy to find studies in highly specialized aspects of psychiatric nursing which are largely irrelevant to the work of most psychiatric nurses. The majority of psychiatric nursing still takes place in mental hospitals, yet there appeared to be little research interest in this less glamorous end of psychiatry. No studies of nursing interventions in relation to chronic institutionalized patients or the elderly mentally infirm could be found. There does appear to be a need to identify priorities for future research.

A range of methods and techniques have been employed by the researchers in this book. These include interviews, self-completion questionnaires, analysis of records, methodological and experimental designs. In an attempt to integrate these diverse studies, comments by the Editor will be found at the beginning of each chapter.

References

Brooking, J. I. (1984). Advanced psychiatric nursing education in Britain. Paper given at the Association of Integrated and Degree Courses in Nursing Annual Residential Conference, University of Sheffield, July 1984.

Marks, I. M., Hallam, R. S., Connolly, J., and Philpott, R. (1977). *Nursing in Behavioural Psychotherapy*. Royal College of Nursing, London.

Paykel, E. S. and Griffiths, J. H. (1983). *Community Psychiatric Nursing for Neurotic Patients*. Royal College of Nursing, London.

Part A   Reviews of Research

CHAPTER 1

A Review of Recent Research in Psychiatric Nursing

Editor's Comments

In this chapter Bryn Davis lays the foundations for the book by reviewing recent British and American psychiatric nursing research. Obviously a short chapter can do no more than point out some areas of interest, identify some key studies, consider general trends and future directions. Bryn Davis also considers some methodological issues and shows how from simple beginnings psychiatric nursing research is becoming increasingly sophisticated and complex.

'. . . we can learn from our mistakes. They develop a theory of knowledge and of its growth.'

(Popper, 1972, p. vii)

Introduction

Trial and error may seem a hackneyed phrase with which to describe the process of knowledge building, of research, of science since it gives the impression of almost accidental discovery. Yet in essence it means testing some idea or conjecture. The result may show error or success, leading to the development of a new idea or suggestion for practice. But can something as simple as this be research, science, the development of knowledge? This chapter is concerned with a discussion and review of research in the context of psychiatric nursing. The first part involves a discussion about knowledge and its relation to research and science from which is developed a consideration of the areas contributing to the knowledge on which psychiatric nurses may draw. The central part of the

3

chapter presents a review of recent research into psychiatric nursing, and this is followed by a brief discussion of where it might properly go from here.

Research and Knowledge

For the purposes of this chapter, I want to identify two types of knowledge: private, personal; and public, institutional. We all possess our own knowledge, which we have slowly acquired during our lives. Some we have borrowed from others (parents, close friends, teachers); other aspects of our knowledge are the result of our own experience, our dealings with the world. The latter are things we have tested for ourselves. It can be argued that we can only really 'know' something we have worked out for ourselves, or have experienced.

Consider the difference between knowing about depression from books, from tutors, from patients and having coped with depression as an individual. The former is public knowledge, the latter is private. Scientific knowledge is essentially shared, public, knowledge. Consequently private, personal knowledge, can become shared and enter the public domain. However, there is more to scientific knowledge than that it is shared. It must also be tested, checked, and validated in other peoples' experience. The scientific method is the process by which such tests or validation occurs, and research is the scientific method in action.

Science, or research, starts from problems, questions, conjectures concerning our experience or anticipation of the situations in which we find ourselves. If we consider the knowledge base on which we practice our nursing to be scientific, research based, it means that it is not just borrowed from other peoples' private knowledge but that it has been tested, rejected, modified, developed. Scientific knowledge is always in a dynamic state of becoming, of growing, of generating new ideas, hypotheses, and of being tested.

The scientific method or research can be seen as a cycle or process. As is shown in Figure 1, the stages of the process lead back to the beginning. Thus our research based practice or discipline develops and grows. It is never complete; there are always more questions, more problems, other ways of seeing things. As Popper (1972) argues there is no one source of knowledge, but the most important one, quantitatively and qualitatively is tradition, example, what is taught. It is from this that questions must arise, ideas must be generated, problems recognized and tackled, if the tradition is ever to become knowledge.

	DEVELOPMENT OF A BODY OF KNOWLEDGE OR THEORIES
which leads to	THE GENERATION OF IDEAS
and	QUESTIONING
and	PROBLEM SOLVING
by	SYSTEMATIC STUDY
using the	SCIENTIFIC METHOD
in	CONTROLLED SITUATIONS
allowing	PREDICTION, REFUTATION, EXPLANATION
and	PROVIDING PATHWAYS OF ACTION
on the basis of	THE BODY OF KNOWLEDGE OR THEORIES
which leads to	THE GENERATION OF IDEAS . . .

Figure 1   Definition or model of research

Research for Psychiatric Nurses

When psychiatric nurses are attempting to practice their profession in the light of public scientific knowledge, where should they seek that knowledge? Which tradition informs them; who is asking the questions; who is generating ideas and testing them? It is possible that the range is wider than most of them imagine. Figure 2 shows schematically the sources

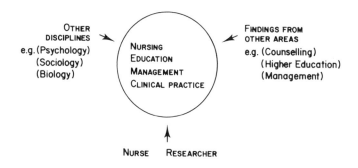

Figure 2   Research and nursing: sources of knowledge

on which educators, managers, and practitioners can draw. On the left is indicated examples of other disciplines, working within the traditions and knowledge of the life sciences, the social sciences, as well as other health care professionals whose work interacts, or could interact with psychiatric nurses. Their questions, problems, and conjectures have a direct relevance to nurses and can have a major contribution to make. Thus we have work by psychologists, sociologists, physiologists, remedial therapists, psychiatrists, perhaps administrators, economists, client groups, which feeds on and directly into the common store. As indicated on the right of Figure 2 there are those whose concerns are not in the least connected with mental health care, but whose way of asking questions, testing hypotheses, challenging tradition can bring inspiration, in spirit or in principle. For example, studies of industrial relations in other service industries, careers guidance, professional training, and higher education.

Finally, however, there are nurses themselves, as indicated at the bottom of the figure. Increasing numbers are now facing up to tradition, challenging and testing what they have borrowed from their mentors, and validating their own and their colleagues' experiences by increasingly rigorous methods. The nature of these methods and the techniques used to ensure as thorough a test as possible of the conjecture or the hypothesis, is a subject which must be dealt with elsewhere. Nevertheless, it is possible to consider the kinds of research being undertaken into psychiatric nursing. The next, central section of this chapter consists then of a review of recent work, with a view to setting the scene for those who wish to follow.

Research into Psychiatric Nursing

There seems to be a surprising amount of research available for consideration. Not only in this country but also in others, particularly the United States of America, psychiatric nursing has generated and continues to generate many research questions. In an earlier review of this material (Davis, 1981) some 65 articles and reports were selected from the period 1972–1979 with the majority being published in the years 1976–1979. By far the majority were projects undertaken by nurses, many of whom were working in the academic field. Less than one third of these studies were concerned with the evaluation of nursing. The vast majority were concerned with identifying or specifying psychiatric nursing.

For the present review, some 33 reports and articles have been collected from the period 1980–1984, with the bulk being published in the years 1981 to 1983. As is shown in Table 1, a wide range of topics has been covered by these reports, the majority being concerned with education. Close runners up are community psychiatric nursing and nurse therapists. Concern for the definition of the nurses' role seems to be concentrated now in these two latter areas, with education being the main general interest. Communication as an area of specialist interest is losing its importance as is behaviour rating. Work on token economy and behaviour therapy is hard to find.

The level of inquiry in the research reports reviewed here is relatively simplistic, in that the majority are overviews or descriptive studies

Table 1 Areas in which psychiatric nursing research has been undertaken in the period 1980–1984

Areas	Number
Nurses' role	4
Nurse education	12
Communication/relationships	3
Nurse therapists	5
Behaviour rating	3
Community psychiatric nursing	6
	33

Table 2 Types of research design used in the literature reviewed

Type	Number
Descriptive studies	10
Correlational studies	5
Experimental	5
Action research	3
Reviews	10
	33

(Table 2). It is important to explain the point of including reviews in this overview. These are papers that have been published as a statement about the current body of knowledge in a particular area. They may be considered as second level research, first level research being research reports themselves. However, many, if not most, research projects involve a preliminary review of the literature in order to establish the credentials of the project being planned. Such reviews consider the most efficacious, creative, important next question arising from the literature; the most feasible, and apt methods and the nature of the results to be expected. Some of these literature reviews are then published separately from the report of the research project. Some of those reviewed here are of this kind. Other reviews are undertaken as an exercise in themselves, or as a dissertation as part of an academic course. This kind is also reported here. Some reports of research are published complete with the literature review, and have not been included in the category Review. Examples of these are Cormack (1983) and Shanley (1984).

Although we still have a major concern to observe where we are now (an essential preparatory phase of any inquiry), a large proportion of the studies reviewed here express a concern with 'why we are here', so to speak. Relationships are sought between facets or variables of our situation. However, only a few are involved with the experimental manipulation of variables in an attempt to test hypotheses.

The smallest group of reports are concerned with action research. Action research involves the monitoring or evaluation of planned change in a particular setting. The results of the evaluation are then reported to those in the setting and any necessary adjustments made to the programme prior to a further period of evaluation. Although it echoes the aims of experimental research, it can rarely achieve the degree of operational control that is necessary. Some action research designs may qualify for the category 'quasi experimental design' (Campbell and Stanley, 1966).

Of the studies reviewed here almost two-thirds are from the United States of America. They are not the only examples of American psychiatric nursing research but they have been selected because they are from the period being reviewed, and they have been published in relatively accessible journals. There are strong arguments against the unquestioning acceptance of research findings from another country. Although English speaking, there are important cultural differences, particularly with reference to psychiatry, between America and Britain. Nevertheless, study of these reports does show how common are some of the questions being raised, and how relevant some of the postulated solutions may be. Much key nursing research has been undertaken in the USA and it is important that we acknowledge this and do not feel that we must start with a clean sheet in every instance. The six areas of psychiatric nursing research will now be considered individually and there will follow a concluding section about the implications of this review for future research and practice.

The Psychiatric Nurse's Role

The work of Cormack (1981, 1983) in the UK offers two major contributions to research in psychiatric nursing. First, and perhaps the most important at the present stage of research, is that of methodological development. In the main study the use of Critical Incident Technique is explored. Attempts to describe social, professional situations are fraught with problems and Cormack has presented some of these in his earlier work (1976). In the most recent study (1983) he demonstrates further consideration of this issue.

Most techniques for collecting information in studies that attempt to fathom the nature of interactions and roles, for example, frequently elicit more information than was intended. In many cases, interviews can extend from information collecting situations to quasi-therapeutic sessions. Cormack's (1981) discussion of the problems encountered with such material is most apt in the light of the increasing number of similar studies. The rigour that is required in survey or descriptive studies, using structured or unstructured interviews, questionnaires or any of the various observation strategies is not always appreciated, particularly by neophyte researchers. Measures to avoid bias or invalidating subjectivity on the part of the researcher are often more noticeable by their absence than otherwise. In his discussions Cormack makes a salutary contribution to this kind of research.

The two American reports in this section show a very different level of concern. Cormack describes a general overview of the psychiatric nurse's role whereas those from across the Atlantic are concerned with very special aspects of that role: crisis intervention in the case of bereavement (Constantino, 1981) and suicide prevention (Fitzpatrick, 1983). The former of these describes a procedure in use but is non-evaluative and small scale. Its value rests in its innovativeness and in the discussions about the role of the nurse and the place for crisis intervention in the armoury of strategies available in psychiatry. The report by Fitzpatrick is a historical review of the study of suicide and its prevention with particular reference to the work of the psychiatric nurse. Exploring different strategies used by the professionals through the varying changes in public as well as professional attitude to this topic, a picture emerges of changes in perceptions of the psychiatric nurse's role. Although much of our concern over the last decade or so in psychiatric nursing research has been with 'where are we now?' (see Davis, 1981), there is an increasing tendency to concentrate on specific aspects of this. In particular this is shown by the number of studies concerned with education which are discussed in the next section.

The Education and Training of Psychiatric Nurses

A substantial body of knowledge is now being generated about the preparation of psychiatric nurses. Its development and progress has been charted by Arton (1981) whose historical review charts the legal and professional processes involved up to 1976. Thus the Salmon Report, Briggs Report, and the NHS Reorganization and the new syllabuses are included in Arton's review.

The picture gained from studies of the experiences of student nurses during training and factors influencing them, such as the programme of research undertaken by the present author (Davis, 1984a,b,c and Chapter 5 in this book) raises questions about ways of improving the relationships between learners and their significant others, as well as the teaching and support available in the clinical setting. Evidence of differing attitudes towards mental health care between the various age groups in the nursing service, the relationship between attitudes and anxiety, and the possibility of influencing attitudes through informal discussion groups has been offered (Davis 1984a,b). Attitudes and responses to training seem to be related to wastage rates and certainly are associated with stresses experienced by learners during their practical experiences. Many report a lack of support and guidance and a great need for self-reliance during their training (Davis 1984c and Chapter 5; Clinton 1981; Powell 1982).

One way of tackling this situation has been suggested by Reynolds and Cormack (1982) and Reynolds (1982). They argue that patient centred teaching, utilizing clinically based teachers, and drawing on a problem-orientated approach to nursing, could greatly facilitate the process of becoming a nurse. Their descriptions of an action research project implementing this new way of educating and training psychiatric nurse learners give graphic illustrations of the potential benefits to be gained. It would seem to be a proposal worthy of further testing in other settings.

Another new development in methodology is Repertory Grid Technique, used by the present author (Davis, 1985 and Chapter 5) and by Wilkinson (1982). This latter study was concerned with the effects of three months psychiatric nursing experience on general student nurses. It was found that anxieties expressed prior to the experience were still present afterwards. The students appreciated certain aspects of psychiatric nursing, in particular the opportunity to talk to patients and undertake assessments of them.

Attempts to evaluate nurse education and training, other than by obtaining the perceptions and reactions of the learners have been few. French (1980) introduced a particular teaching technique (academic gaming) and found it popular with students, as well as effective in increasing knowledge. He also found that the students studied did not value private reading as a learning technique. Squier (1981) attempted to develop a rating scale for the assessment of nurse learners. The results, however, were disappointing, the scale being unreliable and lacking in validity. Raters were influenced by 'halo' effects and a tendency to deal with stereotypes.

Concern with nurses after basic training has been the focus of two studies recently. Coombes and Rana (1981) undertook a follow-up of nurses who had completed an integrated SRN/RMN training course. Most were in clinical posts and many had undertaken further training at post-basic level. It was also found that most nurses were currently employed in the specialism which was their second qualifying course. There was an 18 per cent wastage rate over the period studied. This study highlights the importance of studying the career patterns of nurses and leads to a concern over the opportunities available to them for post-basic education. This was the emphasis of the study by Bridge *et al.* (1981) which was an attempt to survey the kinds of courses validated by the Joint Board of Clinical Nursing Studies and offered by various centres. Generally the findings reveal many difficulties, in funding, staffing, and recruiting for these courses. However, they also demonstrated the potential, particularly in the light of priorities and policies proposed by the Department of Health and Social Security (1981).

These studies of nurse education and training have relevance also to the revelations about the lack of congruity between prescribed and observed roles in psychiatric nursing (Cormack, 1983; Shanley, 1984). The definition of psychiatric nursing roles is of great concern to most people involved in the preparation of nurses at basic and post-basic levels. In the next sections studies of particular aspects of, or developments in, psychiatric nursing roles are presented.

Community Psychiatric Nursing

This is an area where much interest has been shown. Substantial reviews by Sladden (1979) and Parnell (1978), as well as experimental studies by Corrigan and Soni (1977), Davis and Underwood (1976), and Warren (1971) have set the scene for developments in the period under review. A major project has been that by Paykel *et al.* (1982). This study also included extensive discussions of the implications of this role and the need for evaluation (Griffith and Mangen, 1980; Mangen and Griffith 1982a). The main study, a random prospective controlled study was an admirable attempt at the experimental evaluation of community psychiatric nursing (CPN) in comparison with alternative strategies of psychiatric care. No clinical differences were found between CPN care and that provided by hospital psychiatrists at out-patient clinics. However, there were more discharges, fewer referrals to psychologists and more contact with general practitioners (Paykel *et al.*, 1982). The patients found the CPNs more approachable and sympathetic, and were more satisfied. There was some evidence for a cost benefit with the use of CPNs (Mangen and Griffith 1982b).

Hunter (1980) reviewed the literature concerning the CPN role compared with that of the psychiatric social worker, and suggested that these roles should be complementary and that there was a need to avoid the danger of overlap between them. In an observation study of two CPN systems, general hospital based and psychiatric hospital based, Hall and Russell (1982) found the general system led to fewer patients having more time spent on them, whereas with the psychiatric system more patients were seen. They queried whether the general system was meeting the needs of the community in its development into a more specialist service. This is obviously an area of professional role development of major importance and its importance demands that we ask questions of it and rigorously test the assumptions.

Communication

This type of research has been of major concern for British psychiatric nursing since the early work of Altschul (1972). However, it is only represented here by two reports. Macilwaine (1981) described the findings from a series of interviews with nurses and patients in a psychiatric unit in a general hospital. She showed that there was a large discrepancy between their respective perceptions of their interactions. She wondered whether congruence of perceptions might not have therapeutic value echoing questions generated from Altschul's study (1972). Allen (1981) in her report describes the kinds of things nurses talk about among themselves. She found that they talk a lot about their patients. This she suggests provides a function in maintaining the social structure of the unit, as well as some of the personal needs of the staff themselves and their morale.

An American study has concentrated on the importance of non-verbal communication, particularly with reference to the evaluation of empathy in psychiatric nursing, (Hardin and Halaris, 1983). Those nurses expressing high empathy were found to show most non-verbal activity in their interactions with patients. This research generates many more questions about the nature of empathy, its mechanisms and acquisition. The relationships between the kinds of pictures revealed by studies of what nurses say (or do not say) and the information being gained about the emotional 'climate' between staff and between staff and patients are other fruitful areas for study.

Nurse Therapists

Although there have been a few studies in the last decade in the UK describing and evaluating the nurse therapist role and preparation (Davis, 1981), in the period under review the main effort seems to have been in the USA. There the role of nurse therapist has a somewhat wider application than on this side of the Atlantic. The studies being considered are all concerned with attempts by nurses to institute intervention in specific care situations. Fishel and Jefferson (1983) set up a programme of assertiveness training, run by nurses, with a wide range of patients, using experimental and control groups. Significant differences were found between these in terms of scores on the Adult Self-Expression Scale. The strongest effect was observed with depressed patients. Post and Oteri (1983) were also concerned with depressed patients and describe a system of partial hospitalization for those expressing suicidal thoughts or intentions. These two studies show clinical and management initiatives being taken by psychiatric nurses. The study by Whiteside (1983) in a quasi-experimental design attempted to evaluate an educational programme instituted by the nursing staff to inform patients about their medications, the kinds of drugs involved, the effects to be expected, and the nature of prescriptions. Significant differences were observed between experimental and control groups in terms of pre- and post-test knowledge.

In these latter studies the emphasis seems to be more on nursing interventions, whereas in the UK the emphasis would be most associated with a psychotherapeutic role. One report from the USA is concerned more with this aspect, being a review of recent work on Milieu therapy (Devine, 1981). In the UK Strang (1982) has described and discussed the psychotherapist role, with particular reference to drug dependency. A 'friend' role and a 'therapist' role were identified, and the skills needed in shifting from one to the other when necessary, discussed. Unfortunately there are neither details of the kind of interviews undertaken nor of the preparation or evaluation.

The differences between American and British perceptions of nurse therapy reflect differences in approaches to the psychiatric nursing role. In America there is much more interest in problem orientated approaches to care, to assessment of need, planning interventions, and evaluating outcomes. The next and final section in this review considers recent studies that attempt to assess behaviour in an attempt to evaluate care.

Behaviour Rating

The need to assess carefully the nature of the psychiatric nursing need prior to the planning of a suitable care programme has inspired attempts to develop instruments to facilitate this. Capodanno and Targum (1983) review previous work in the assessment of suicide risk and describe briefly proposals for a new rating scale. No evaluation is offered but the need for it is acknowledged. In the area of child psychiatry, Webb et al. (1983)

in a quasi-experimental design, report the evaluation of a structured paediatric psychosocial interview schedule. Experienced and inexperienced raters were used and it was found that both groups produced consensus rating, in that inter-rater reliability between and within the groups was high. No other forms of evaluation were reported. Important questions as to the clinical validity of both of these instruments are raised and provide impetus for further research.

In the UK concern with the evaluation of good psychiatric nursing has been shown by Shanley (1984). Reviewing the literature he finds the discrepancies between the prescribed and described role of the psychiatric nurse. Developing his own rating scale, Shanley describes his first attempts to validate this through comparisons between ratings by charge nurses and patients of the same nurses, and also by comparisons with other scales. Although the results are somewhat inconclusive, they confirm the importance of such work, and generate further research questions into this whole area.

Conclusions

From a period covering almost five years, a range of psychiatric nursing research reports have been presented and described, all too briefly. Although the subject matter has been most varied, a few major categories have been identified. Within these it can be seen that many questions are being asked by psychiatric nurses, even such basic ones as 'what is?'. Attempts to describe psychiatric nursing are initiated by the conjecture that there are parameters, or there is a structure, a process that can be revealed by suitable techniques. Research skills involve the selection or creation of methods which will test these assumptions.

In many ways the sophistication of attempts to develop a body of scientific, public knowledge is revealed in the armoury of techniques available. An important trend in psychiatric nursing research can be seen in the development or utilization of an increasingly rigorous range of research designs and methods. An important aspect of the reports reviewed here has been the description of research techniques, new, or relatively new, to psychiatric nursing. These have been highlighted in the previous sections but can be usefully mentioned here again. The Critical Incident Technique used by Cormack (1983) already has a substantial pedigree and from this research report it would seem to offer scope for many more investigations. When offering a picture of a process or a system, for which there can be many varying interpretations or perceptions, the use of this technique as an anchor or a constant from which to consider the constructions offered, is a major advance on the more ephemeral material all too frequently obtained from interviews. The combination of this technique, with observational data supported by video or cine recording, is a further refinement which can increase the rigour with which the questions, conjectures, and assumptions are tested.

Repertory Grid Technique is another addition to the range of methods available. Already established in the fields of clinical psychology and educational psychology, it is now being utilized in psychiatric nursing. When the questions or conjectures concern relationships between elements of the situations involving nurses, patients and the delivery of care, it offers an opportunity to evaluate idiographic or group data. Essentially devised as a way of demonstrating how individuals view their world, or aspects of it, and channel their actions with respect to it, it is a technique with great potential for monitoring the effect of innovation, therapy, education, and counselling, particularly in the Situational Dependency Grid format (Davis, 1985).

As well as the range of techniques available to test hypotheses or conjectures, however, the choice of research question is perhaps the most important. Most psychiatric nursing research consists of unrelated, small scale studies although the quality of the literature reviews being produced now is pulling together these small scale studies to produce a relatively consolidated body of knowledge. Nevertheless, the choice of what to research next can be difficult.

In the United States attempts have been made to develop programmes or policies of coordinated research which reflect the development of the body of knowledge. This has been done for the study of organizations, by psychologists, for example, and for psychiatric nursing. In both cases 'expert opinion' was recruited to determine priorities. The psychologists, who were commissioned by the Industrial and Organisational Division of the American Psychological Association, sent a special survey form to 200 registered members of the Division (Campbell *et al.*, 1984). These selected members, including a preponderance of current researchers, were each asked to nominate up to six important research needs. One hundred and five replied and their suggestions were subjected to a content analysis, using a set of categories derived from an analysis of current research. A wide range of suggestions resulted, demonstrating that the 'experts' did not have a well-worked out view of what they wanted to do. There was relatively little consensus. General comments, however, were made by the authors. Many of the respondents complained of a lack of practicality in current research, and of its elitist nature. There was also a concern expressed about the difficulty in producing the full answer to questions into which much research energy had already been invested. The authors were concerned at the generality of many of the research suggestions which made them essentially unanswerable. They also acknowledged that the lack of consensus and the generality of the suggestions may be related to the format of the survey.

A development in the method of determining lists of priorities which attempts to produce more of a consensus view is the Delphi technique. This is the technique used in the survey of priorities of psychiatric nursing research referred to above (Ventura and Waligora-Serafin, 1981). It was developed in the 1950s and has been used in a variety of settings in order to determine priorities based on expert opinion. The special development offered by this method is that once having elicited a range of topics for study, and having these categorized by a panel of experts, the list of statements defining the categories is returned to the respondents for rating. They are asked to re-rate them according to their impact on the care of patients. These ratings are then analysed and median scores for each statement obtained. These results are then returned to the participants who are asked to re-rate the statements in the light of the median scores provided with them. From this second round of ratings the list of priorities is generated.

Ventura and Waligora-Serafin (1981) surveyed both general and psychiatric nurses and have reported separately the results from the latter group. The highest rated items included factors contributing to repeated hospital admissions; the role of the nurse in continuity of care after discharge from hospital; patient compliance; the contributing factors to staff 'burnout' (an American term used to describe the collapse of the spirit indicated by disillusionment, lacklustre performance, and a preoccupation with impersonal aspects of nursing, if not by withdrawal from the role). Others contained reference to the effects of hospitalization, prevention of suicide, care planning, patients' readiness to learn, care of terminally ill patients, mental health maintenance, and quality nursing care. Of the fifteen highest rated items, the majority were introduced by the words 'define' or 'explore'. A minority (five) were concerned with evaluation, although four more asked for the development of criteria, which would lead to evaluation and assessment. This approach to the planning of research, to the establishment of priorities for policy making, is also occurring in the UK. A survey of randomly selected nurses in Scotland, including psychiatric nurses, is being planned, using the Delphi technique (Nursing Research Unit, 1983). This follows the example of Bond and Bond (1982) in the North East of England, but with attempts to overcome some of the methodological problems highlighted in the latter study.

Such attempts to develop strategies for research by making public the shared priorities of those concerned can be seen as part of the process of making research relevant to the practitioner. This is also important for those who fund research. Most of those who implement research, and those who support it, require that research that is undertaken is seen to be making meaningful contributions. But whose opinion as to the relevance of research priorities is most valid? The survey of psychologist experts is of a different order from that undertaken by Ventura and Waligora-Serafin (1981) where practitioners, not researchers or academics, were questioned. There are important issues to be raised here. Should the research that is undertaken be guided and generated by the knowledge, the theory that already exists, or by the kinds of solutions required by those who apply that knowledge? Is practice based on the public scientific knowledge or on individual private knowledge? Is the public knowledge or theory relevant to the needs of the practitioners?

In psychiatric nursing it seems that we are beginning to realize the importance of developing a public scientific knowledge base or theory on which to base our practice. We are also incorporating and developing in our research techniques and methods which enable us to test more rigorously the questions, hypotheses or conjectives that arise. What is also important, however, is that we begin to incorporate this public knowledge in our own personal knowledge and practice.

References

Allen, H. (1981). 'Voices of concern' — a study of verbal communication about patients in a psychiatric day unit. *Journal of Advanced Nursing*, 6 (5), 355–362.

Altschul, A. (1972). Patient–nurse interaction; a study of interaction patterns in acute psychiatric wards. Churchill Livingstone, London.

Arton, M. (1981). The development of psychiatric nursing education in England and Wales. *Nursing Times*, 77, January 15th, 124–127.

Bond, S. and Bond, J. (1982). A Delphi survey of clinical nursing research priorities. *Journal of Advanced Nursing*, 7 (6), 565–576.

Bridge, W., Dunn, P., and Speight, I. (1981). The provision of post-basic education in psychiatric nursing. *Nursing Times*, 77 (52), suppl. 36, 141–144.

Campbell, D. T. and Stanley, J. C. (1966). Experimental and Quasi-Experimental Designs for Research. Rand McNally and Co. Chicago.

Campbell, J. P., Daft, R. L., and Hulin, C. L. (1984). What to study; generating and developing research questions. Sage, London.

Capodanno, A. E. and Targum, S. D. (1983). Assessment of suicide risk. *Journal of Psycho-Social Nursing*, 21 (5), 11–14.

Clinton, M. E. (1981). Training psychiatric nurses. A sociological study of the problem of integrating theory and practice. Unpublished PhD thesis, East Anglia University.

Constantino, R. E. (1981). Bereavement crisis intervention for widows in grief and mourning. *Nursing Research*, **30** (6), 351–353.

Coombes, R. B. and Rana, S. C. (1981). An integrated SRN/RMN course. I and II. *Nursing Times*, **77**, suppl. 16 April, 45–48; 23 April, 49–52.

Cormack, D. F. (1976). *Psychiatric Nursing Observed*, Royal College of Nursing, London.

Cormack, D. F. (1981). Making use of unsolicited research data. *Journal of Advanced Nursing*, **6** (1), 41–49.

Cormack, D. F. (1983). *Psychiatric Nursing Described*, Churchill Livingstone, Edinburgh.

Corrigan, J. and Soni, S. D. (1977). Community psychiatric nursing: an appraisal of its impact in community psychiatry in Manchester. *Journal of Advanced Nursing*, **2**, 347–354.

Davis, A. J. and Underwood, P. (1976). Role function and decision making in community mental health. *Nursing Research*, **25**, 256–258.

Davis, B. D. (1981). Trends in psychiatric nursing research. *Nursing Times*, **77** (19), occasional paper, 73–76.

Davis, B. D. (1984a). Student nurse wastage and attitudes to treatment. *Nurse Education Today*, **4** (4), 89–91.

Davis, B. D. (1984b). Student nurse attitudes; their modification and associations. *Nurse Education Today*, **4** (5), 117–120.

Davis, B. D. (1984c). Interviews with student nurses about their training. *Nurse Education Today*, **4** (6), 136–140.

Davis, B. D. (1985). Dependency grids: applications in education, in N. Beail (Ed.), Repertory Grid Technique and Personal Constructs. Croom Helm, Beckenham, Kent.

Department of Health and Social Security (1981). *Care in Action*, HMSO, London.

Devine, B. A. (1981). Therapeutic milieu/milieu therapy: An overview. *Journal of Psycho-Social Nursing*, **19** (3), 20–24.

Fishel, A. G., and Jefferson, C. B. (1983). Assertiveness training for hospitalised emotionally disturbed women. *Journal of Psycho-Social Nursing*, **21** (11), 22–27.

Fitzpatrick, J. J. (1983). Suicidology and suicide prevention. *Journal of Psycho-Social Nursing*, **21** (5), 20–28.

French, P. (1980). Academic gaming in nurse education. *Journal of Advanced Nursing*, **5** (6), 601–612.

Hardin, S. B. and Halaris, A. L. (1983). Non-verbal communication of patients and high and low empathy nurses. *Journal of Psycho-Social Nursing*, **21** (1), 14–20.

Hunter, P. (1980). Social work and community psychiatric nursing — a review. *International Journal of Nursing Studies*, **17**, 131–139.

Griffith, J. H. and Mangen, S. P. (1980). Community psychiatric nursing — a literature review. *International Journal of Nursing Studies*, **17**, 197–210.

Hall, V. and Russell, O. (1982). The Community Mental Health Nurse: A new professional role. *Journal of Advanced Nursing*, **7** (1), 3–10.

Macilwaine, H. (1981). How nurses and neurotic patients view each other in general hospital psychiatric units. *Nursing Times*, **77**, July 1, 1158–1160.

Mangen, S. P. and Griffith, J. H. (1982a). Community Psychiatric Nursing Services in Britain: The need for policy and planning. *International Journal of Nursing Studies*, **19** (3), 157–166.

Mangen, S. P. and Griffith, J. H. (1982b). Patient satisfaction with community psychiatric nursing: A prospective controlled study. *Journal of Advanced Nursing*, **7** (5), 477–482.

Nursing Research Unit (1983). *Annual Report*. Nursing Research Unit, University of Edinburgh, 12 Buccleuch Place, Edinburgh.

Parnell, J. W. (1978). *Community Psychiatric Nurses*. An abridged version of the report of a descriptive study. Queen's Nursing Institute, London.

Paykel, E. S., Mangen, S. P., Griffith, J. H., and Burns, I. P. (1982). Community psychiatric nursing for neurotic patients: A controlled trial. *British Journal of Psychiatry*, **140**, 573–581.

Popper, K. R. (1972). *Conjectures and Refutations*. Routledge and Kegan Paul, London.

Post, J. M. and Oteri, E. M. (1983). Sign-out rounds. *Journal of Psycho-Social Nursing*, **21** (9), 10–17.

Powell, D. (1982). Learning to Relate. Royal College of Nursing, London.

Reynolds, W. (1982). Patient centred teaching: A future role for the psychiatric nurse teacher. *Journal of Advanced Nursing*, **7** (5), 469–475.

Reynolds, W. and Cormack, D. F. (1982). Clinical teaching: An evaluation of a problem orientated approach to psychiatric nurse education. *Journal of Advanced Nursing*, **7** (3), 231–237.

Shanley, E. (1984). How psychiatric nurses are seen by their charge nurses and their patients. Unpublished PhD thesis, University of Edinburgh.

Sladden, S. (1979). *Psychiatric Nursing in the Community: a Study of a Working Situation*. Churchill Livingstone, London.

Squier, R. W. (1981). The reliability and validity of rating scales in assessing the clinical progress of psychiatric nursing students. *International Journal of Nursing Studies*, **18** (3), 157–169.

Strang, J. (1982). Psychotherapy by nurses — some special characteristics. *Journal of Advanced Nursing*, **7** (2), 167–171.

Ventura, M. R. and Waligora-Serafin, B. (1981). Study priorities identified by nurses in mental health settings. *International Journal of Nursing Studies*, **18**, 41–46.

Warren, J. (1971). Long acting phenothiazine injections given by psychiatric nurses in the community. *Nursing Times*, **67**, 141–143.

Webb, T. E., Adams, M. R., and Van Dere, C. A. (1983). Listening reliably to psychosocial concerns of youth. *Journal of Psycho-Social Nursing*, **21** (6), 25–28.

Whiteside, S. E. (1983). Patient education: effectiveness of medication programs for psychiatric patients. *Journal of Psycho-Social Nursing*, **21** (10), 16–21.

Wilkinson, D. (1982). The effects of brief psychiatric training on the attitudes of general nursing students to psychiatric patients. *Journal of Advanced Nursing*, **7** (3), 239–253.

CHAPTER 2

Undergraduate Research in Psychiatric Nursing

JULIA BROOKING

Introduction

All final year students of the Bachelor of Science (Honours) degree in Nursing Studies at King's College, formerly Chelsea College, University of London, undertake a research project as part of the degree requirements. This small scale study is carried out over about four full-time months and each student is supervised by a lecturer in the Department of Nursing Studies. Students are free to select any area or method of study, as long as it is related to nursing. Some of the students choose to carry out psychiatric nursing projects.

The main part of this chapter contains an outline description of previously unpublished research in psychiatric nursing carried out by students at Chelsea College between 1981 and 1984. This includes an account of aims, methods, and findings, as well as some discussion of the implications and limitations of the studies.

The final part of the chapter is a critical examination of the scope, range, advantages, and problems of undergraduate research in psychiatric nursing. The chapter concludes with an assessment of the contribution of undergraduate research to psychiatric nursing knowledge and indicates some suitable areas for further study.

Outline Description of Students' Projects

Ros Alstead (1981).
Relatives of psychiatric patients: a consideration of the degree of information and support they receive from psychiatric nurses.

21

Aims

The study aimed to examine the extent to which relatives wanted information and support; whether they were provided; nurses' beliefs about giving information and support to relatives; and the extent to which relative involvement was encouraged by medical and nursing staff.

Methods

Semi-structured interviews were carried out with 27 registered nurses on admission wards in one psychiatric hospital. Fifteen relatives of patients admitted for the first time to one psychiatric hospital were interviewed.

Results and discussion

The data were analysed in terms of three themes as now described.

Involvement of relatives Most relatives claimed they were not involved, but most nurses claimed that opportunity for involvement was available if they were interested. Relatives who were involved claimed they had to ask questions and seek advice. Nurses encouraged relatives to visit but did not use visits as opportunities for counselling or exchange of information. Alstead argued that the nurses' approach was purely patient-centred and that their training did not equip them to respond to relatives' needs for reassurance, support, and information.

Exchange of information Relatives wanted information to increase their understanding of the patients' problems but this need was not met. Many nurses feared that giving detailed information would infringe the doctor's role. Alstead recommended that ward policies were needed to ensure the provision of information to decrease family stress. At the time of admission relatives wanted information about the functioning of the ward to reduce their anxiety. Seventy-five per cent of relatives reported receiving very little information on admission but 66 per cent of nurses said that detailed information was given. Nurses were found to initiate interactions rarely and largely for their own benefit. When questioned by nurses, relatives rarely knew why they were being questioned. Nurses assumed that if relatives wanted information they would ask, yet the evidence suggested that relatives who were most in need of support and guidance felt least able to ask for it.

Impact of admission on relatives Mental illness and admission had a considerable impact on the psychological well-being of the relatives, causing family disruption, shame, stigma, social withdrawal, and attempts at concealment. Nurses were seen as having the greatest understanding of their problems and being easiest to talk with.

Recommendations

Alstead recommended that more attention should be given to relatives' needs and that nurses should be trained to respond to relatives' fear, anxiety, and family disruption. She argued that the establishment of a key worker could reduce the problems.

Limitations of the study

The study used only one hospital and had a small sample, so should not be widely generalized. No clear hypotheses were formulated as the study was intended as pilot work to aid the formulation of specific hypotheses. The use of semi-structured interviews creates a problem in obtaining a balance between richness and quality as compared with precision and objectivity. Comparison of the data from nurses and relatives was complicated as nurses had to generalize, whereas relatives described specific experiences.

Karen Jones (1981).

Psychiatric illness amongst an immigrant population: a comparison of referral methods, length of stay in hospital, and disposal methods of two selected groups admitted to Springfield Hospital during 1979.

Aims

The study aimed to identify how a person's culture could affect referral to, length of stay in, and discharge from a psychiatric hospital.

Methods

Case records of patients admitted to and discharged from one psychiatric hospital in 1979 were examined. From a total of 324 records, the records of 56 immigrant patients (West African and West Indian) were matched with the records of 56 English-born patients for age, sex, diagnosis, and occupation.

Results

There was little difference in the referral agencies used by the two groups but reasons for referral differed. A larger proportion of the immigrants presented with disturbed behaviour, whereas more English patients than immigrants presented with suicide attempts and depression. The duration of symptoms before admission was shorter for the English sample, but the immigrants had a shorter length of stay in hospital than the English sample. On discharge a large proportion of both groups returned to their former lodgings, but more of the English sample were rehoused. The immigrant sample had less previous contact with the psychiatric services before 1979, but more readmissions over that year than the English sample.

Limitations of the study

It would be unreasonable to draw conclusions from such a small study carried out in one hospital. The results may be attributable to random differences among groups. Patients were not matched for the number of previous admissions, which is another uncontrolled variable. Using records as a source of data permits bias in various ways. The staff who recorded information were mostly English-born, which may have biased their understanding of the immigrants' problems, which should be considered within their cultural context. The diagnosis of 'disturbed behaviour', for example, begs more questions than it answers. The researcher's expectations may have biased her interpretations of the data, especially as the subjects' cultural group was known to the researcher. It is almost impossible to check the validity of case-record data and the patients' own perceptions of their problems are not available.

Kath Unwin (1981).

A case study to investigate problems faced by nurses on a psychogeriatric ward.

Aims

The study aimed to investigate the work of nurses in one psychogeriatric ward; in particular to examine nurses' attitudes to work and their perceptions of problems in the provision of care; to examine what work on the ward involved; and to study the demographic characteristics of staff and patients.

Methods

This descriptive study used natural observation in an uncontrolled setting without manipulation of variables. One ward was studied intensively using informal interviews, activity studies, short questionnaires, and observation. Non-participant observation was initially planned but some participation became essential to gain acceptance from staff.

Results and discussion

There were 41 patients in the ward with a mean length of stay of 6 years and 9 months. Most had no prospect of discharge. The average age of the men was 67 and of the women was 77. Seventeen per cent were always incontinent, 46 per cent were sometimes incontinent, 15 per cent were immobile, 24 per cent had no rational conversation, and 46 per cent had fragmentary conversation. Most of the patients were diagnosed as suffering from senile dementia, but a few were 'burned out' psychotics. Thirteen nurses worked on the ward, four registered, five enrolled, and four auxiliaries. There were no learner nurses as the ward was not approved for nurse training. An activity study of the nurses' time showed that basic care occupied 28 per cent of their time, 25 per cent of the time was unoccupied, 13 per cent of the time was meal breaks, 10 per cent was clerical work, 7 per cent was technical care, mainly feeding patients, 7 per cent was serving meals, and the remaining time was spent on dealing with linen, medicines, stores, and administration. The nurses' day typically involved 'tremendous onslaughts' of physical care, followed by long periods away from patients, sitting and relaxing. The ethic of the ward was to get the work done quickly and then relax, which was one reason why nurses liked working there. The nurses perceived their problems to be (in rank order): a shortage of staff, insufficient time for psychological care, lack of equipment, wandering patients, and lack of understanding by senior staff. Unwin observed that nurses' conversations with patients tended to be affectionate, teasing, and bantering. They occurred randomly and had no planned therapeutic content. Unwin argued that the lack of systematic psychological care was not due to lack of time, but to a lack of training in psychological aspects of care and interpersonal skills. Most patients were forced into dependent roles, irrespective of their actual needs.

The nurses expressed a general lack of confidence in senior staff. Unwin argued that there was a need for more contact between nurses at ward level and in management, and for involvement of nurses in decision-making if improvements in standards of care are to be seen.

Limitations of the study

Although the ward was selected as a typical psychogeriatric ward, the results should not be generalized. This method does not permit checking of the data or replication, so researcher bias is a strong possibility. The presence of the observer on the ward may itself have influenced practices, at least for the first few days of the study.

Clare G. Street (1982).

An investigation of the priority on nurse–patient interaction by psychiatric nurses.

Aims

Recent psychiatric nursing literature has emphasized that high priority should be placed on interpersonal relationships and nurse–patient communication. This study aimed to identify nurses' actual work priorities, the factors that influenced their priorities, and whether they accorded with the priorities identified in the literature.

Methods

Twelve qualified and trainee nurses in three acute admission wards of one psychiatric hospital were observed for a total of 97 hours. The researcher observed two nurses at any one time, in a non-participant capacity and using time sampling checklists. Following the observations the twelve nurses were interviewed using a semi-structured schedule. Pilot studies were carried out.

Results and discussions

Subjects' ranking of various nursing activities showed that nurse-patient interaction was generally given high priority whereas routine or physical care activities were ranked as less important. However, the researcher observed very little correlation between the priorities expressed in the interviews and observation of the actual work. Routine administrative tasks appeared to be most important and a high proportion of the day was spent in the ward office. One staff nurse complained that much of the paperwork could be done by a clerk. Street observed that time for nurse–patient interactions was not structured into the day. Only if and when routine activities were completed did nurses have the opportunity to talk with the patients.

There were great individual differences in the amount of time spent talking with patients, but on average nurses spent two and a half times more time in the ward office than with patients. Not surprisingly, nurses who said they placed low priority on communicating with patients spent most time in the office. One nurse was observed to spend a whole shift without talking individually to any patient. The least experienced nurses (four first-year students) spent on average 24 per cent of their time talking with patients, whereas the more senior nurses spent only 14 per cent of their time on average talking with patients.

Street considered that although more than half the nurses recognized in theory that interacting with patients should be a high priority, in practice this was rarely achieved. She concluded that these nurses were not active members of the therapeutic team as advocated in the literature.

Limitations of the study

The general problems of observational studies discussed in relation to Unwin's work are applicable here, such as the influence of the observer on subjects' behaviour, the representativeness of the period observed, the risk of observer bias and lack of replicability. The presence of a second observer would have allowed some check on inter-rater reliability and would have increased confidence in the findings. The sample was very small and subjects were not randomly selected. The sample contained nurses of different grades: pupils, students, and staff nurses. Although some interesting differences among groups emerged (e.g. pupil nurses were the only subjects who ranked physical care as top priority), the numbers in each grade were too small to permit meaningful comparisons.

H. Louise Toms (1982).

The role of registered mental nurses: custodians or therapeutic agents?

Aim

The study aimed to examine whether there were any differences in custodial and therapeutic attitudes and care between nurses working in a therapeutic community and traditional admission wards of a psychiatric hospital.

Methods

The researcher designed a Likert-type scale which measured attitudes towards custodial care (7 items) and towards therapeutic care (14 items). Subjects responded: strongly agree, agree, disagree or strongly disagree to each item. Examples of themes included in the custodial subscale were the nurse being in charge of the patient; the patient being dependent on the nurse; patients being excluded from ward meetings, etc. Examples of themes included in the therapeutic subscale were patients participate in care planning; nurses discuss patients' feelings; nurses are involved in therapy groups etc. Sixteen registered mental nurses completed the scale, of whom six worked in a therapeutic community (response rate six out of seven) and ten worked in traditional admission wards in a large psychiatric hospital (response rate ten out of thirteen).

Results

Nurses in the therapeutic community were all under thirty-five and two-thirds were single. In the traditional admission wards a third of the nurses were over thirty-five and two-thirds were married. There were also differences between the types of patients in the two areas. Many patients in the therapeutic community were suffering from neurotic and personality disorders, whereas more patients in the admission wards suffered from psychoses and depression.

Toms used the Mann Whitney U test to examine differences between the two groups of nurses. Nurses in the therapeutic community had significantly higher mean scores on the therapeutic scale than nurses in the traditional admission wards ($p < 0.05$) and significantly lower mean scores on the custodial scale ($p < 0.01$). The overall scores of the nurses in the traditional admission wards had a higher standard deviation, that is they were more variable than the scores of the nurses in the therapeutic community which tended to be closer to the mean. This suggests a greater diversity of attitudes in the admission wards. Nurses who wore uniforms had significantly higher scores on the custodial scale than those who did not wear uniform. There were no differences among subjects according to gender, age, marital status, qualifications (RMN only or RMN and SRN), and length of employment.

Discussion and limitations of the study

It appeared that nurses in the therapeutic community tended to have more therapeutic and less custodial views than nurses in the traditional admission wards. However, constraints of time and resources prevented the researcher from testing her questionnaire for validity and reliability, so no firm conclusions should be drawn from the study. Many of the nurses trained in the same school of nursing, which suggests that differences in attitudes might be attributable to the work environment, although attitude differences could account for choice of work environment in the first place. Information about the choice these nurses had in selecting their work place would have been useful. The sample was very small and the analysis was limited, both of which further reduce the validity of the findings. The lower standard deviation in the scores of nurses in the therapeutic community was an interesting finding. Paradoxically, the therapeutic community may have demanded conformity to the prevailing ethos of the community, whereas the traditional admission wards may have been more permissive in accommodating a greater diversity of opinion.

Carol Usher (1982).

Attitudes towards mental illness: a comparative study of student psychiatric nurses and student general nurses.

Aim

The study aimed to examine whether experience of nursing those with mental illness affected nurses' attitudes to it.

Methods

The researcher compiled a six-point Likert type attitude scale from previously used questionnaires, of which 16 items indicated positive attitudes towards mental illness and 16 items indicated negative attitudes. The subjects were 29 psychiatric nursing students and 31 general nursing students prior to any experience of psychiatric nursing. A convenience sample of students in study block at the time of the project was used. All students were members of the same school of nursing.

Results

Using the Mann Whitney U test, Usher found several statistically significant differences between the two groups. The RMN students obtained higher overall scores showing more positive attitudes to mental illness than SRN students. SRN students were more rejecting of the mentally ill than RMN students, for example larger numbers thought the mentally ill should not be allowed to have children, did not see them as ordinary people, would be ashamed to be mentally ill themselves, and thought it was easy to see the difference between mentally ill and normal people. The SRN students felt more sorry for mentally ill people than RMN students and expressed more fear and embarrassment about mental illness. The RMN students expressed more positive, accepting, and humanitarian attitudes towards mental illness than SRN students, were more tolerant of the mentally ill in the community, and were more knowledgeable about the legal status of mentally ill patients admitted to hospital. The general nursing students expressed similar attitudes to those of the general public as found in a study by Maclean (1969).

Discussion and limitations of the study

The researcher concluded that psychiatric nursing students expressed more positive attitudes towards many aspects of mental illness than general nursing students. It may be that experience of working with the mentally ill produced more positive attitudes, but it is likely that before beginning training the RMN students had more positive attitudes which influence their career choice. A serious problem with the study was lack of matching between the two groups. The psychiatric nursing students were in the third year of training, were mostly aged 23 to 27, and included men and women. The general nursing students were in the first or early second year of training, were mostly aged 19 to 21, and were all female. Any of these differences may have accounted for the results. The attitude scales were not thoroughly pretested and no estimates of validity and reliability were obtained.

Sarah M. Mobbs (1983).

Liaison between nurses and other occupational groups in a psychiatric hospital.

Aims

The number of occupational groups involved in hospital psychiatric care has proliferated in recent years, so nurses have an important role as overall coordinators of care. It is therefore important that nurses understand the roles of other team members and are able to liaise effectively with them. This study aimed to investigate:

1 nurses' knowledge about the work of other occupation groups;
2 nurses' knowledge of referral methods and obtaining advice from other occupational groups;
3 how other occupational groups expect to be contacted by nurses and whom patients and relatives ask for information about available facilities;
4 whether responses varied according to the type of ward and seniority of nurses.

Methods

Data were collected in one psychiatric hospital. Postal questionnaires were sent to two or three members of each of 16 occupational groups selected by a panel as important to hospital care. These included social workers, occupational therapists, ministers of religion, clinical psychologists, psychiatrists, voluntary workers, dietitions, etc. Structured interviews were carried out with 70 nurses ranging in seniority from auxiliaries to nursing officers, 25 patients, and 16 relatives. The nurses, patients, and relatives were drawn from admission, long stay and psychogeriatric wards, and day care.

Results and discussion

An interesting finding was that over half the members of the various occupational groups thought that nurses should have sufficient knowledge of their function to continue in their absence activities that they had initiated. Similarly, nearly a third of the patients and relatives thought that nurses should continue with the treatment of other occupational groups in their absence. This raises several questions. Firstly, does training adequately prepare nurses for this multiplicity of roles? Mobbs argued that it did not, as nurses' knowledge about the roles of other team members was generally poor, especially among auxiliaries, learners, and enrolled nurses, and among nurses in long stay and psychogeriatric wards. Secondly, should nurses function as assistants to all other mental health workers? This problem is particularly associated with multidisciplinary team care in which nurses often occupy low status and subservient roles. It seemed paradoxical that over half the members of other occupational groups would not accept patient referrals from nurses despite expecting nurses to be able to continue their work in their absence.

Patients, relatives, and members of other occupational groups clearly expected nurses to act as liaison figures, but frequently claimed that nurses did not fulfil this function adequately. Relatives and patients relied heavily on nurses for information about other occupational groups, yet their needs for information were often not satisfied. Mobbs concluded that better teaching in this area and improved communication between nurses and other occupational groups were essential for effective liaison and coordination of care.

Limitations of the study

This study described practices in just one large psychiatric hospital and it is not legitimate to assume that the same results would be found elsewhere. The sample was small, largely self-selected, and somewhat imbalanced. No patients from psychogeriatric wards were suitable to take part, no relatives could be found in long stay wards, and many qualified nurses refused to take part. The rather complex design produced a mass of unwieldy data, which were analysed only descriptively. Inferential statistics were not used because of the small numbers in the subgroups. The questionnaires and interview schedules, although pilot-tested, were not examined for validity or reliability.

Joanna C. Bune (1984).

The role of the community psychiatric nurse in the prevention of mental illness.

Aims

This study aimed to investigate the role of the community psychiatric nurse (CPN) in the prevention of mental illness. It specifically aimed to discover: the extent to which a sample of CPNs were involved in preventive activities, how much their education prepared them for the role, and the views of CPNs and related psychiatric professionals towards the role of the CPN in prevention.

Methods

Each CPN in one hospital-based service ($n = 16$) recorded their work activities for a week on specially designed forms, after which they were interviewed. Samples of nurse managers ($n = 5$), psychiatrists ($n = 5$), and psychiatric nurse tutors ($n = 5$) were interviewed. All CPN course senior tutors in England were sent questionnaires and six out of ten responded. All instruments were pilot-tested.

Results

Eighty-one per cent of the CPN sample were engaged in the primary prevention of mental illness according to their work sheets. However, this activity occupied only 19 minutes a day on average. Factors which reduced their ability to engage in preventive work were said by the CPNs to include (in order of frequency) the type of referral system, lack of time, bureaucratic factors, lack of training, and lack of literature. Half the CPNs believed their education prepared them for a preventive role; but none of the CPN course senior tutors believed that CPNs were adequately prepared for prevention; and 60 per cent of psychiatric nurse tutors believed that pre-registration learners did not receive sufficient education in this subject. Of the total sample, only a third were convinced that it was possible to reduce the incidence of new cases of mental illness. Of the total sample 72 per cent thought CPNs had a role to play in primary prevention, 89 per cent in secondary prevention, and 92 per cent in tertiary prevention. This indicates that secondary and tertiary prevention were seen as more important roles for CPNs and only 8 per cent of the total sample thought that primary prevention was a more important role for CPNs.

Discussion and limitations of the study

The study demonstrated that this group of CPNs did have a role in the prevention of mental illness, but it was limited by various factors, of which the most important seemed to be the system of referral from consultants to whom the CPNs were attached. Bune argued that the key to increased CPN involvement in preventive work lies in their attachment to primary health care teams, working with clients who have not been diagnosed as mentally ill. The sample was small and only one hospital-based CPN service was studied, both of which factors limit the generalizability of the findings.

Discussion Of Undergraduate Research In Psychiatric Nursing

The eight small studies summarized in this chapter have produced some interesting and unexpected findings, with many implications for practice, and, perhaps more importantly, they have generated numerous ideas for larger scale research.

Ros Alstead (1981) identified problems experienced by patients' relatives, their needs for information and support from nurses and the inadequacy of current nursing interventions with relatives. These findings point to the opportunity for expansion of the psychiatric nursing role to help distressed and anxious relatives. Karen Jones (1981) identified some areas of possible differences between English born and Afro-Caribbean psychiatric patients, which suggest topics for further study in large, carefully controlled and preferably prospective studies. Kath Unwin (1981) provided an insight into the work of nurses in a psychogeriatric ward and highlighted problems such as lack of attention to patients' psychosocial needs. She identified some reasons for these difficulties, such as nurses' sense of powerlessness in decision-making, lack of support from managers, and lack of continuing education for these nurses. Clare Street's (1982) study drew attention to the discrepancy between nurses' awareness in theory that talking with patients is important and their actual work in admission wards, where talking with patients occupied little time and was given low priority. Two studies of nurses' attitudes produced unsurprising results. Louise Toms (1982) found that nurses working in a therapeutic community expressed more therapeutic and less custodial attitudes than nurses working in traditional psychiatric admission wards. Similarly, Carol Usher (1982) found that psychiatric nursing students expressed more positive attitudes towards mental illness and mentally ill people than general nursing students, prior to a psychiatric placement. Sarah Mobbs (1983) identified ineffective communication and conflicting expectations between nurses and other mental health workers. Patients and relatives also expressed dissatisfaction with the ability of nurses to liaise between patients, families, and other psychiatric professionals. Joanna Bune (1984) confirmed the view that prevention is part of the work of community psychiatric nurses, but that organizational factors such as referral methods inhibited the development of this role.

An examination of the eight studies as a group reveals several themes in the results which suggest further research. Several studies implicate inadequate education as a possible contributor to deficient practice. Topics which could be included in post-basic education, as suggested by these results, include the development of skills for communicating with patients, relatives, and colleagues, the roles of other team members, psychological needs of special groups of patients, such as the elderly and the needs of relatives. Studies to evaluate the effectiveness of post-basic education in terms of skills, knowledge, and attitudes would be feasible and might lend support to further educational developments. Another theme to emerge from these studies is the lack of information and counselling given by nurses to patients and relatives. Studies of the effects of various types of information and counselling interventions on a range of outcomes such as psychiatric symptoms, treatment compliance, anxiety, participation in care would be interesting and valuable. Another way of improving nurse–patient relationships may be by introducing systematic care planning and the allocation of individual nurses to specific patients. Such innovations in nursing practice could be evaluated on a variety of measures.

Undergraduate research makes an important contribution to research training and instills enthusiasm in many students to carry out larger postgraduate studies. Students have demonstrated understanding of and profiency in a wide range of research methods and techniques including structured and semi-structured interviews, self-completion questionnaires, attitude measurement, participant and non-participant observation, and retrospective analysis of case records. Other psychiatric nursing projects not included in this chapter have used methodological and historical designs. Experimental designs are not usually feasible.

Methodological problems associated with undergraduate research are illustrated by this selection of studies, many of which have common limitations, despite being carried out at different times and supervised by different lecturers. Inevitably the studies have small samples and are usually carried out in one hospital. They tend to be over-ambitious, attempting to examine several factors and producing unwieldy data, which the students are unable to analyse fully.

There is generally inadequate pretesting of instruments developed by the students, such as attitude scales and questionnaires. This problem is so common that it can be argued that students should either collect data using well-established instruments, or they should carry out methodological work to develop and test an instrument. It is difficult to do both in the time available.

Other methodological problems include the lack of linkage among studies and the lack of replication. Each student tends to start with an entirely new topic. Increasingly, students are advised to work in pairs on closely related topics. Because of time constraints these projects inevitably have to examine what already exists, rather than introduce and evaluate new practices. Consequently the studies nearly always produce criticisms of existing practices, which may seem negative and threatening to nurses reading about them.

There can be conflict concerning the aims of the studies. Are they intended as educational exercises for research training or can they produce meaningful results? The ideal answer is that the studies aim to do both, but in reality students vary in their ability to produce valid and useful results. This dilemma is associated with an ethical question. If the studies are mainly educational, can the use of valuable staff time which would otherwise be devoted to patient care be justified? Equally, is it justifiable to involve patients and their families who are already distressed by the illness? These are complex questions about which students should be individually advised according to their chosen area of study, their ability, and personality. It can be argued that some patients enjoy and even benefit from participation in non-invasive nursing research, because of the attention they receive, their interest in the topic, and their desire to contribute to nurses' education and the development of knowledge. Nurses may also benefit from direct contact with research by being stimulated to examine their own practices, by reading the results, and by developing an awareness of the relevance and importance of research.

The final area of difficulty concerns access to the research site. Although proposals have been approved by an ethical committee, there has been a marked reluctance by some psychiatrists to allow patients to participate in studies. Some doctors react negatively to the development of psychiatric nursing as an academic and research-based discipline and indicate that they regard research by nurses as unnecessary and even dangerous. It is the responsibility of nurses to ensure that psychiatrists understand developments in psychiatric nursing practice, education and research, the aims of which are the improvement of patient care, not the take over of medical functions. In recent years senior nursing staff have been helpful in facilitating access and have expressed interest in the work. However, many ward-based nurses have refused to participate, especially qualified nurses in long-stay and psychogeriatric wards. Perhaps they feared that inadequate practices would be revealed, or perhaps they regarded the studies as time-consuming and pointless. This attitude creates a real risk that developments in psychiatric nursing research will be blocked by psychiatric nurses themselves. There is clearly still a long way to go in educating psychiatric nurses about research.

Reference

Maclean, V. (1969). Community attitudes towards mental illness in Edinburgh, *British Journal of Preventative and Social Medicine*, **23**, 45–52.

Note The projects described in this chapter were submitted in part fulfilment of the BSc (Honours) Nursing Studies degree at Chelsea College, University of London. Copies of the dissertations are lodged in the University of London libraries at King's College and St George's Hospital Medical School.

Part B   Psychiatric Nursing Education

An Examination of the Psychiatric Nursing Component of Degree/RGN Courses in Britain

EIMEAR MUIR-COCHRANE

Editor's Comments

Eimear Muir-Cochrane's study arose from this Editor's concern as a newly appointed nursing lecturer that there was little shared information about how psychiatric nursing was taught in other British nursing degree courses. Psychiatric nursing lecturers in universities and polytechnics work mainly with general nursing lecturers and seem rather isolated from psychiatric colleagues. Eimear Muir-Cochrane attempted to obtain information about the psychiatric nursing component of general nursing degrees in England, Scotland, and Wales. She sent postal questionnaires to all course tutors and gave self-completion questionnaires to students from six such courses. This chapter will be of particular interest to anyone concerned with psychiatric nursing education at undergraduate level.

Introduction

All nursing degree courses include some education in psychiatric nursing, but the content and organization of this part of the degree varies widely. This study examined the psychiatric nursing component of degree/RGN (Registered General Nurse) courses at universities and polytechnics in England, Scotland, and Wales. Northern Ireland was excluded for personal reasons.

The aims of the study were to collect information about psychiatric nursing courses from teachers and students in order to:

1   compare courses at each college, identifying differences and similarities;
2   assess the effectiveness of courses for their clinical and educational value;
3   give course planners an insight into students' perceptions of courses;
4   enable course planners to share the experiences of colleagues in other colleges;
5   provide information which could be used to improve psychiatric courses.

Postal questionnaires were sent to the lecturers/tutors in charge of psychiatric nursing education in each of the fourteen degree/RGN courses and twelve were returned completed. Questionnaires were also completed by eighty-eight undergraduate student nurses in six colleges offering various types of degrees with RGN. All the students had completed a psychiatric nursing course.

This study provides for the first time a picture of the way psychiatric nursing is taught to and experienced by degree/RGN students in England, Scotland, and Wales. Implications for nursing education and practice and recommendations for improvements are also discussed. The work was carried out between October 1982 and May 1983 as part of the author's degree requirements (Muir-Cochrane, 1983).

Review of the Literature

In the field of psychiatric nursing there is an increasing demand from nurses to be recognized as therapists in their own right. However, there is little evidence to suggest that psychiatric nurses play an active therapeutic role in the care of their patients and their nurse training prepares them better for a 'monitoring role than an active role' (Cormack, 1976). Mitchell (1976) believes that there is a great disparity between standards of educational experience available to undergraduate and RGN nurses. The reasons for this are complex and require detailed study.

Mitchell (1976) and Pattermore (1966) emphasized the importance of orientation and preparing general nursing students for their psychiatric experience. This would also help in improved staff/patient communication and a higher level of discussion within the nursing team. Ujhely (1968), Rodger (1972), and Jourard (1971) found a lack of emotional and psychological awareness by nurses of patients needs. There was little encouragement by their tutors/ward staff to have such awareness or realize its existence.

Arton (1981) describes the development of degree courses incorporating psychiatric nursing from 1969 and the NHS reorganization which brought syllabus changes. In 1976 Emblin and Hill described the various existing degree courses in nursing. However, the only research associated with degree nursing and psychiatric courses was by Denny and Denny (1979) who compared the UK Mental Health Programmes with psychiatric components of Baccalaureate programmes.

It is obvious from this brief review that further investigation is warranted in the fields of psychiatric nursing experience within degree courses and psychiatric nursing education itself.

The Method of Study

The Lecturers' Questionnaire

The lecturers' questionnaires with explanatory letters were sent to the lecturer in charge of the psychiatric nursing course at each of the fourteen university and polytechnic nursing departments in England, Scotland, and Wales. The questionnaires consisted of open ended and closed questions to gather data on areas such as length of the course, whether compulsory or optional, theoretical and clinical content and balance, clinical setting, who runs the course, opinions of the course, and opinions of what students learn from the course. The questionnaires had previously been pilot tested on two lecturers. The data were analysed to discover trends and characteristics of the course, difficulties encountered with the course, and to form a comprehensive report of psychiatric components of degree/RGN courses throughout the country.

The following are typical examples of the questions included:

1   How long in days is the psychiatric experience including both clinical and theoretical components?
2   Is the course fragmented (e.g. 1 day/week) or continuous (e.g. a two-month period)?
3   Is the psychiatric course run by:
(a)   nursing department of university/polytechnic,
(b)   hospital school of nursing,
(c)   others,
(d)   combination of (a), (b), and (c) (please describe)?

The Students' Questionnaire

A separate self-completion questionnaire was given to a sample of eighty-eight undergraduate student nurses at six colleges, five in the London area, and one in the provinces; all the students had completed their psychiatric placement. It was hoped that students' perceptions of the course would be discovered and could be related to staff perceptions. The following are typical examples of questions used:

1   Describe which aspects of class teaching were most helpful in looking after patients on the wards.
2   Which of your teachers gave you the most relevant information?
(a)   hospital school of nursing tutors,
(b)   university or polytechnic nursing lecturers,
(c)   ward staff,
(d)   psychiatrists,
(e)   others.
Please explain your choice.

The sample was a total population of nursing students who attended a particular lecture on a certain date and were invited to fill in a self-completion questionnaire. Fifteen to twenty questions were used to gather information about the students' attitudes to psychiatric nursing and mental illness, the balance of clinical and theoretical work, and enjoyment or stress experienced during the course.

   The study of students' opinions was retrospective, as they had completed the psychiatric experience between four months and two years before filling in the questionnaire. Although this is a limitation the data reflect the important issues since students only remembered their outstanding feelings of the time. All the students were verbally informed in detail by the researcher about the aims and purpose of the study. Although cooperation was invited they were assured that there was no obligation to take part.

Response Rates

Response rates of students filling in questionnaires was very good. Only eight out of eighty-eight students declined to fill in the questionnaires. Reasons given for non-compliance were lack of time and lack of interest in the project. Only two lecturers' questionnaires out of fourteen were not returned completed. Reasons for non-return are unknown. Therefore the response rate from students was 93 per cent and from lecturers 86 per cent.

Analysis of Results

Quantitative data were analysed using frequency tables, percentages, and other descriptive statistics. Inferential statistics were not used as the data were inappropriate. Qualitative data were analysed by modified content analysis to categorize comments. Tables were also used to illustrate differences between the twelve courses studied. Table 1 is an example of how qualitative data from a Lecturer's Questionnaire was tabulated.

Table 1 Tabulation of qualitative data

Institution	Chelsea College (London University)
Length of course	40 days
Form of course	Continuous eight-week block
Time of year	June/July
Responsibility of course	*Mainly school of nursing with contribution from university nursing lecturers
Existence of introduction to course	*One day in first week in school of nursing
Wards involved in students clinical experience	*Short stay (long stay if requested but only for two weeks)
Do students have a choice of ward?	*Yes—can choose to work for two weeks elsewhere after six weeks on short stay
Type of shifts when nursing	Early/late shifts, no weekends, no night duty
Number of classroom days	Nine days, one study day a week, one introductory day
Formal organized lectures given by:	*School of nursing tutors, psychologists, community psychiatric nurses, psychologists, university nursing lecturers
Do specific objectives exist?	Yes
Are these realized by students?	*No
Existence of formal assessments	Ward sisters report, university nursing lecturer's report—*written exam set and marked by school of nursing tutors, care study
Contribution to overall degree class	*Does not count towards degree but must be satisfactorily completed

*Now changed

The psychiatric nursing course at Chelsea College became an examined part of the degree from summer 1984. Students' clinical and academic work for the course now counts towards the final degree class awarded.

A Discussion of Findings from Lecturer and Student Questionnaires

There are two main ways of obtaining an RGN qualification with a degree: integrated degrees and combined degrees. The former degree entails the student being based in a university/polytechnic department and obtaining a degree in nursing. The latter entails obtaining a degree in a subject related to nursing while separately studying for the nursing qualification in an associated hospital. Psychiatric nursing experience is a compulsory element in both types of degree courses, but performance in most courses does not count towards the final degree class.

Course Organization

In general, psychiatric courses in integrated degrees are organized by psychiatric nursing lecturers in universities/polytechnics, whereas in combined degrees psychiatric nursing is usually taught by nursing tutors based in the school of nursing.

The designation of this responsibility depends on the following kinds of factors: the existence of lecturers within the nursing department, qualified in psychiatric nursing to organize such a course; the form of liaison with psychiatric hospitals in that area and access for degree students to complete a psychiatric experience there. Finally, if the RGN students' psychiatric experience is seen as suitable and appropriate for the degree nursing students then the nursing department would accept hospital tutors organizing the course. However, the standards of education, support, and guidance are not always acceptable in their existing form so alternatives need to be provided.

Course Content

The courses varied considerably in length and academic and clinical content. The length of courses varied from 18 to 56 days. Mean length was 36 days. Students expected to work on some of the following areas: acute/admission ward, psychogeriatric ward, behavioural therapy unit, day hospital, specialized/general and medium/long stay wards.

Introduction to the courses lay in the form of community experience, lectures, and orientation days. At one college the school of nursing tutor responsible for the course remarked that no formal introduction existed, and 'introduction by practical experience' was the only valuable form of introduction. All courses contained theoretical and clinical teaching but no general standard existed and some courses appeared to be more fragmented than others. The nursing students worked normal or modified early/late shifts but no night duty.

Course Objectives

It became apparent from results that school of nursing tutors were not aware of evaluation of the course objectives although they recognized their existence. This may have been due to poor communication between the tutors and university/polytechnic lecturers. The nursing tutors also often lacked information about the purposes of the courses, students' previous academic and clinical experience, and how the psychiatric course slots in to the degree as a whole.

Commonly expressed aims and objectives included gaining insight into the care of the mentally ill and the role of the nurse, understanding treatments and medication, developing interpersonal skills, and the assessment and identification of problems related to mental health and associated legislation.

Satisfaction and Dissatisfaction with the Course

There exists some disparity between views of hospital tutors and university/polytechnic lecturers. Generally hospital tutors were more satisfied with the courses than lecturers. Aspects of the courses which lecturers and tutors found satisfying were the opportunity to do classroom and clinical teaching; contact with students and facilitating student/patient relationships.

Dissatisfaction was expressed about the shortness and timing of the courses, predominance of the medical model and poor standards of care with insufficient good role models for students. Generally hospital tutors commented much more positively and less critically about teaching by ward staff than university/polytechnic lecturers.

Students found satisfaction in interacting therapeutically with patients in a relaxed, non-hierarchical atmosphere. Dissatisfaction lay in the lack of systematic care planning on the wards, boredom, carrying out menial tasks, and the emphasis on the medical model.

Students' Attitudes

Students' comments regarding attitude change during the courses focused on insight gained from the experience to see patients as ordinary people. They generally felt less apprehensive about looking after patients and more sympathetic and confident in doing so.

Fifty-eight per cent of lecturers/tutors thought that nurses' attitudes had altered after the experience. Comments suggested that students gained a broader more informed view of mental health. It was also felt that negative attitudes developed towards the ward staff, their norms, and their values. Overall, lecturers and tutors expressed the view that it was not the fact that attitudes had altered (or not altered) that was important, but the insight they had gained in this area where stigma and criticism prevail.

Teaching by Lecturers/Tutors

Students claimed dissatisfaction with any teaching using the medical model. Aspects seen as valuable were case history discussion, the use of coping mechanisms, behavioural aspects, and communication skills. Aspects not covered that students felt would have been useful were the work of Szasz, counselling, the care of overdose patients, and general under- or misinformation.

They called for improvements in method and form of such teaching, utilizing more discussion groups of smaller size and a shift away from the medical model of treatment. They expressed a need for a theoretical experience that would help them on the wards, utilizing knowledge gained in the classroom.

Students gave a mixed response about whether lecturers, tutors or others gave the most relevant information. This raises the interesting question as to whether those organizing the experience are expected to give the most relevant information or is their role to organize other people to do so.

Ward-based teaching

Teaching by ward staff covered topics such as rehabilitation, community care, the Mental Health Act, and planning and implementation of care. However, students complained that this teaching was given on an informal almost accidental basis during report or if students asked for more information. Students gave a very mixed response to the actual usefulness of this teaching but did recognize its existence. However, a small number of students stated that they had received no teaching at all. This is an important point because it may mean that, depending on the wards worked on, some students could receive a lot of very useful information and others none at all.

Students called for more teaching from nursing rather than medical staff and more guidance when caring for patients. They expressed a need for structured teaching sessions at specifically arranged times and maximizing the use of report as a teaching session. Lecturers, too, were critical of the quality and quantity of teaching that students had received from ward staff but tutors commented favourably about this. Tutors emphasized the importance of practical experience and skills: skills that apparently could not be learnt anywhere except on the wards.

Summary of Questionnaire Findings

The existence of a disparity between hospital tutors' interpretations, views and expectations of the course and of degree students, and those of university/polytechnic lecturers has been discovered. Role definition seems to be lacking so that a 'woolly' idea exists of what hospital tutors should expect from degree students, what the students' aims are, why they are doing the psychiatric course, and what they should gain from it. There also seems to be little clarity in how these tutors provide a suitable experience for the students when they have little factual knowledge about the different degree courses as a whole, and at what stage of the four-year courses students are undertaking the experience.

Fewer problems are seen to exist where the university/polytechnic lecturers run the psychiatric course. Alterations to courses play a large part in providing an experience that is useful and essential to students' experience within the whole degree course. At Liverpool, Surrey, Hull, and Chelsea such changes are under review. These reviews must be persistent and progressive.

Students are noted to have recognized and acknowledged all useful and relevant aspects of the courses while being constructively critical in suggesting alternative methods. Their motivation and assertion is apparent. Many of their suggestions for improvement in ward and class room based teaching parallel comments by lecturers, and student and lecturer perceptions seem to be at least in some way equivalent. In the light of students' comments it must be obvious that organizers of such courses should modify psychiatric experiences for the benefit and satisfaction of all involved.

Critique of the Study

One limitation of the project lay with the nature and design of the questionnaires. Three questions were misinterpreted and so results in those areas were lacking. If more time had been available the questionnaire could have been further refined by more extensive testing for validity and reliability.

Ideally undergraduate nursing students from all twelve courses should have completed questionnaires, since the views of students from six courses, five of those in London, may not necessarily be representative of the views of degree student nurses as a whole.

Overall, the questionnaire to students was found to be, in practice, rather long and time-consuming to complete (about twenty to twenty-five minutes) and demanding of their memories and motivation. Ideally students should have filled in the questionnaire immediately on completion of their psychiatric course, but due to limited time this was impossible. Students' memories were therefore heavily relied upon, often requiring recall of up to a year. It was difficult to analyse all the descriptive data from the questionnaire but the aim of giving lecturers an insight into their students' perceptions and comparing students' and lecturers' views on the same topic was achieved successfully.

One final limitation of the project was that two very different types of degree courses were being investigated, the integrated degree and the combined degree. The overall picture may have been confused by these two, different and separate types of courses: however it was found that there is no general standard among psychiatric components of either degree type.

Conclusions

It has become apparent that some major differences exist between university/polytechnic and hospital school of nursing run psychiatric courses. The courses have no clearly defined general standard.

The presence of associated and integrated degree nursing courses and their differences has been discussed. However, even amongst degrees in Nursing/RGN courses many different approaches exist and these too need to be recognized and understood in future research.

Most of the psychiatric components have no examination that is integrated into the actual degree. This fact also needs to be examined since lecturers are now calling for a recognized status of this component as part of the whole degree course. This raises the question of whether psychiatric nursing is included in the RGN/degree course simply because it is required by the statutory authorities, or is it recognized by its very unique nature as being important and vital for nursing students to experience? Also, when is it most useful for students to experience care of mentally ill patients? Do students need to have a basis of practical experience and theory or could they gain more from it if it occurred very early in the course, although they would be practically inexperienced? These questions need to be answered with further research.

Another important fact that has come out of this project is the need for support for both lecturers/tutors and students during psychiatric experiences since it is recognized as being both challenging and stressful. Research literature has shown that support reduces the stress, apprehension, frustration, and helplessness sometimes felt by students undertaking care of psychiatric patients.

The gradual impact of the nursing process seems to have highlighted potential difficulties for patients and nurses alike within this field. Boundaries between professionals are becoming increasingly blurred particularly as nursing roles are becoming diversified. Modern psychiatric nursing care must recognize and critically examine these vital issues to advance this Cinderella service and create standards of professionalism within it. To this end psychiatric nursing courses must be carefully assessed, planned, evaluated, and modified where necessary; and nurse educators must seek to create environments in which students can optimally gain experience.

References

Arton, M. (1981). Development of psychiatric nursing education in England and Wales. *Nursing Times*, **77** (3), 124–127.

Cormack, D. (1976). *Psychiatric Nursing Observed: A Descriptive Study of the Work of the Charge Nurse in Acute Admission Wards of Psychiatric Hospitals.* Royal College of Nursing, London.

Denny, E. and Denny, J. (1979). A comparison of mental health nursing education in the UK and the psychiatric component of a baccalaureate programme in the USA. *Journal of Nursing Education*, **18** (1), 42–49.

Emblin, R. and Hill, M. J. (1976). Degree courses in nursing 1, 2, and 3. *Nursing Times Occasional Papers*, **72** (40), 141–144; **72** (41), 145–148; **72** (43), 149–152.

Jourard, S. (1971). *The Transparent Self.* Van Nostrand, New York.

Mitchell, W. (1976). Psychiatric module in general training. *Nursing Mirror*, **142**, 55–56.

Muir-Cochrane, E. (1983). An examination of the psychiatric nursing component of degree/SRN courses at Universities and Polytechnics in England, Scotland and Wales. Unpublished BSc dissertation, Chelsea College, University of London.

Pattermore, W. R. (1966). The value of psychiatric nursing training to the general nurse. *Nursing Times*, 18 March, 382.

Rodger, B. P. (1972). Therapeutic conversation and posthypnotic suggestion. *American Journal of Nursing*, **72** (4), 714–717.

Ujhely, G. B. (1968). What is realistic emotional support? *American Journal of Nursing*, **68** (4), 758–762.

CHAPTER 4

A Pilot Study of Nurses' Attitudes With Relation to Post-Basic Training

KEVIN GOURNAY

Editor's Comments

Kevin Gournay examined changes in nurses' attitudes as a result of undertaking various post-basic nursing courses. He found that the groups varied considerably on a range of measures. Trainee nurse therapists were the least conservative and favoured a more psychological, less organic approach to treatment than psychiatric nurses generally. This finding contradicts the traditional notion of the behaviour therapist as mechanistic and lacking humanitarian qualities. Students on the Developments in Psychiatric Nursing course also differed from psychiatric nurses generally, suggesting that the course may preach to the already converted.

Kevin Gournay's chapter is methodologically interesting as he describes a range of attitude measures which may have relevance to other studies. The chapter illustrates methods for measuring changes in attitude, which may be an important aspect of the evaluation of nursing courses.

Introduction

This study was prompted by two distinct sets of influences. Firstly, the author has been involved in the new short course, Developments in Psychiatric Nursing (English National Board (ENB)) Clinical Course No. 953 and became aware that many of the nurses on the course were attempting to question, and more often than not, change attitudes to their job. Most of these nurses had spent their entire nursing careers in large traditional psychiatric hospitals and hoped to gain from the course, not only new knowledge, but a fresh perspective. It therefore became clear that some sort of measure was essential to defining the attitudes of the students and to assess the impact of the course on these. Thus it was hoped that the results of this study would aid the course planning team to design a curriculum in keeping with course objectives.

The second influence was the experience of the author, who had finished training as a nurse therapist in 1977, and who has worked as a practising behaviour therapist since that time. He had become aware that, more often than not, the term behaviour therapy implied, to many professionals, an approach which was simplistic, mechanistic, and lacking in the humanitarian qualities of the insight oriented approaches. Examples of these misperceptions are common, and other nurse therapists report similar experiences. O'Leary (1984) has reviewed the image of behaviour therapy in a most authorative way, and his findings confirm the author's impressions that public and professional impressions of behaviour therapy differ radically from the actual practice and outcomes.

Thus, it seemed important to investigate the attitudes to psychiatric/ psychological treatment by nurse therapists before and after training. It was felt that objective information about attitude change would clarify the issue of the 'personal style' of the nurse therapists involved. Further, the systematic use of measures of attitude seem an important way of evaluating nurse education, and it was hoped that such measures could be extended over various modes of post-basic training.

Specific predictions of how the attitudes of the two experimental groups would change are set out below, together with details of experimental design and method. Before examining these issues the general literature relating to the study is reviewed.

Review of the Background Literature

Attitude has been studied as a psychological phenomenon since the late nineteenth century and for some time social psychology was virtually synonymous with the study of attitudes. During the mid part of this century the conceptualization of attitude became more complex. For example, Krech and Crutchfield (1948) defined attitudes as 'An enduring organization of motivational, emotional, perceptual and cognitive processes with respect to some aspect of the individual's world'. This trend culminated in Rosenberg and Hovland's (1960) classical description of attitude as a three-component system (i.e. that attitude is composed of three categories of response to attitude objects: affective, cognitive, and behavioural). Recently there has been a trend to viewing attitude again in a unidimensional fashion. Ajzen and Fishbein (1980), for example, distinguish clearly between beliefs, attitudes, intentions, and behaviour. These authors have defined each of these concepts, and described their interrelationships in their scholarly theory of Reasoned Action. This theory has had wide and notable effects on, for example, family planning behaviour, voting in general elections, and changing the behaviour of alcoholics. The measurement of attitude has followed a parallel course in the oscillation between a uni- and a multidimensional view. Further, there has been a consistent observation that attitude itself does not predict behaviour, and as Ajzen and Fishbein (1980) point out, in order to predict behaviour accurately, other variables have to be taken into account. With regard to this specific point, Shanley (1981) has argued that behavioural correlates of attitude have been a notable omission in research. Shanley also points out in the same review article that most research into staff attitudes towards mental disorder has been carried out in the USA.

Caine and Smail (1968) devised an Attitudes to Treatment Questionnaire (ATQ) for psychiatric staff, including nurses. Over the years this measure and a battery which evolved from it (Caine et al., 1981 and 1982) have provided the only systematic means of measurement in this area. The original measure was criticized by Shanley (1981) on the grounds of lacking behavioural correlations and sampling errors. Trauer (1977) used the original ATQ with a group of 191 patients with other measures and subjected the responses to a principal components analysis, and in effect suggested that only the first component of the scale be used. Independently, the scale authors reached this conclusion and thence devised the new battery. This new battery answers some of Shanley's criticisms in that an integral part of the 1982 study is the relationship of battery scores with treatment outcome. Further, the authors have collected more extensive and objective data in validating the new measures.

In essence, this research described the attitudes of a wide range of professionals of differing orientations and followed groups of patients through therapy. They studied the characteristics of responders and non-responders to differing modes of psychiatric/psychological treatment and from their data elaborated their theory of 'Personal Styles' (of therapist and patient) and their implications for patient selection for modes of treatment. The source book and manual give data on a variety of professional groups, some of which is reproduced below.

Hall (1974) used the ATQ in a study of student psychiatric nurses having three months behaviour modification experience. He found that attitude did not significantly change over that period but that nurses scoring highly on conservatism seemed to be more detached from their patients and favour a more organic approach to patient care. Hall concluded that the requirements of nurses in a therapeutic community are not dissimilar to those in a behaviour modification programme. He also called for more sophisticated outcome criteria such as the Critical Incident Technique (described by Ryback, 1967) in a paper on nurse selection.

Milne (1984) has followed the line of Hall's (1974) suggestions and used a wide battery of measures of attitude, skill, and learning in assessing 65 qualified psychiatric nurses undertaking an in-service course in behavioural techniques. Milne found that ATQ scores correlated significantly with previous behaviour therapy experience and that such experience seemed to impair further learning of behavioural strategies.

Recently there have been other attempts to look specifically at small subgroups of patients and staff. Jones and Galliard (1983) looked at attitudes to elderly psychiatric patients and Brooker and Wiggins (1983) at nurse therapists with relation to patient outcome. Brooker and Wiggins used analysis of variance and factor analysis to demonstrate a wide range of therapist performance. They have argued cogently for a more rigorous examination of therapist variables to aid selection, and in this area attitude batteries would obviously be of value when used with other measures.

The literature indicates the need for studies of nurses in various settings using multiple measures, of which an attitude battery would be an obviously useful component. This is particularly true of expensive training such as the ENB Course 650 (Adult Behavioural Psychotherapy) and of new courses such as ENB 953 (Developments in Psychiatric Nursing). The current study is thus a pilot attempt to look at the specific issue of attitude before launching a fuller, more comprehensive study.

Method

It was decided to investigate changes in attitude over training using the five measures detailed below on two main groups, i.e. nurses training as Nurse Therapists on ENB course No. 650 and nurses undertaking the new ENB course No. 953, Developments in Psychiatric Nursing. It seemed reasonable to use another course as a control group, and therefore because of its nature and local availability, ENB course No. 941, Nursing Elderly People, was chosen. Other control courses were considered (e.g. intensive care) but as the chosen course has a more general psychological flavour, it was thought that the questions on the attitude scales would have some relevance for the respondents. Further, while the psychological status of the patient is considered of central importance, this course makes no overt attempt to change attitudes to psychiatric or psychological treatment, although of course such changes may occur incidentally. Thus such a control course would yield valuable test re-test data.

The inclusion of the group of trained nurse therapists as a fourth (reference) group was decided as it would be of obvious interest to see just how the trainee nurse therapists compared. In view of the limitations of such a pilot study it seemed reasonable to only use the two main measures of the study, i.e. the ATQ and the DIQ (Direction of Interest Questionnaire), which have a reasonably well-defined relationship to the other measures.

Thus the battery was given to course members immediately before and immediately after training. As this was a pilot study, no follow-up was planned. In a fuller research project evaluating attitudes, currently being planned, a follow-up would be included, together with the use of behavioural measures such as those used in the Milne (1984) study. This method was clearly outside the scope of the current study.

Subjects

Subjects were drawn from the four groups of nurses, described below.

Nurse Therapist trainees taking ENB Course No. 650
Adult Behavioural Psychotherapy

A complete group of nine trainee nurse therapists at the Maudsley Hospital were chosen and they were assessed immediately before and after training. This training was inaugurated in 1972 and has been described in many sources of literature, including other chapters in this book. The most comprehensive description of the course and its content is to be found in the book by Marks *et al.* (1977). Briefly, the course trains psychiatric nurses to be autonomous case managers with neurotic patients, using a behavioural approach. Training is based on an apprenticeship model, and in all training centres it is conducted in settings where the prevailing treatment philosophy is virtually exclusively behavioural. Selection procedures for this course tend to be lengthy, often over two full days, but there are no formal measures of attitude to treatment used in any of the centres. There are many applicants for this course and successful applicants come from a wide range of settings. Experience post-RMN training, varies from a few months to several years. At the time of the study about 80 nurses had completed the training. One male trainee refused to take part in the study for reasons that were not clear but complete data were obtained from the other trainees.

Nurses taking the ENB Course No. 953
Developments in Psychiatric Nursing

The first two groups of nurses undertaking the course at Napsbury Hospital were chosen and were assessed immediately before and after training. The first group contained 10 students and the second group 11 students.

This course is run for RMN trained nurses with at least 4 years post registration experience and the main aim is to enable nurses to study recent developments and trends in psychiatric nursing. The course explicitly sets out to help nurses focus on their own clinical nursing practice and to consider alternatives. The course provides a Briefing Day, four 5-day intensive blocks of study, and 9 days of practical experience (5 days with community nursing teams and 4 days with a psychologist or nurse therapist observing behavioural procedures). This is all during a 19-week period. The study blocks include up-to-date information on various organic and psychological approaches, together with practical experience of dynamic groups. Apart from this, current nursing practices including the Nursing Process are examined in detail and project work between study blocks is encouraged. This work commonly takes the form of planning and implementing a comprehensive nursing programme with a 'difficult' patient. The psychological treatment orientation of the course organizers and planning team is probably best described as 'eclectic'. The range of post-registration experience in the two groups was 4 to 20 years (mean 9.55, S.D. 4.74).

All 21 course members returned data pre-training and 20 returned data post-training. One course member emigrated before the second rating point.

Nurses taking the ENB course 941: Nursing Elderly People

A complete group of 15 nurses undertaking the course at Barnet General Hospital were chosen and were assessed immediately before and after training. This course aims to help registered and enrolled nurses from a variety of work settings (including general and psychiatric hospitals and community services) to study developments in the care of the elderly and refresh both skills and knowledge. An entry requirement is that nurses should normally have at least two years experience caring for the elderly. The course is spread over a period of approximately 20 weeks (maximum 26 weeks) and comprises 22 study days divided into blocks. As in the course Developments in Psychiatric Nursing, projects relevant to clinical work play an important part. All 15 course members returned data pre- and post-training.

Trained Nurse Therapists:
Graduates of the ENB Course No. 650
Adult Behavioural Psychotherapy

At the time of the design of the study there were 70 practising trained nurse therapists. As this was only a pilot study it was decided to survey half of these. Further, it was envisaged that the other half would be included in a later study using the same questionnaires. Therefore 35 nurses were chosen, using random number tables, and questionnaires posted. Thirty sets of data were returned. There were no reasons elicited for the non-response of the five subjects.

These nurses had been nurse therapists for a mean of 3.3 years (S.D. 2.12, range 1–9 years) and mostly worked as clinicians, although three taught behaviour therapy and one was working in an administrative capacity. They also came from all three training centres. An analysis showed no differences between respondents trained at different centres on questionnaire scores (a fourth centre in Sheffield has yet to produce its first graduate).

Measures

Attitudes to Treatment Questionnaire

The ATQ (Caine *et al.*, 1982) measures staff attitudes to psychological and psychiatric treatment. The scale is said to differentiate between a physical, organic, and impersonal approach to patient care and the more psychological approach characterized by therapeutic communities. As with the TEQ and DIQ (see below) this questionnaire was validated on a large sample of various groups of professionals working in a wide range of settings. Within the nursing groups a wide range of psychiatric nurses was represented (from specialized therapeutic communities to traditional psychiatric hospitals).

Lillie (1973) has concluded that the questionnaire may be considered to distinguish between two broad approaches, namely a psychological and an organic approach. No significant relationship between scores and sex has been found. Milne (1984) found some evidence that the ATQ may be related to age. The scale also has high test-retest reliability. High scores represent a physical, organic approach to patient care, low scores represent a psychological approach.

Table 1   Mean scores on the ATQ for various nurse and doctor samples. Data
reproduced by kind permission of Caine, Smail, Wijesinghe, and Winter (1982)

Specialized therapeutic Community nursing staff	31.83 S.D. 5.68
Group of psychiatric nurses attending a conference	51.18 S.D. 10.65
Nurses from three traditional psychiatric hospitals	62.60 S.D. 10.82
General hospital nurses	61.72 S.D. 7.51
Doctors orientated towards therapeutic communities	37.23 S.D. 7.00
Doctors orientated towards group psychotherapy	48.80 S.D. 7.05
Doctors orientated towards organic approaches	54.17 S.D. 6.41

*Group of 77 nurses from Napsbury Hospital
  (training centre of nurses undertaking
  ENB Course No. 953, Developments in Psychiatric Nursing)
	53.46
	S.D. 12.25

*From Winter et al., (1984).

Treatment Expectancy Questionnaire

The TEQ (Caine et al., 1982) was originally devised to measure patients'
expectancies regarding treatment and in particular differentiates between
preference for medical/behavioural treatments or for group psychotherapeutic treatments. As expectancy is not a static phenomenon test-
retest reliability was not established. No significant sex differences were
found during validation but there is a relationship between high scores
and age. High scores represent preference for medical/behavioural
treatments, low scores for group psychotherapeutic treatments.

Direction of Interest Questionnaire

The DIQ (Caine et al., 1982) is a distillation of three scales of three
personality and vocational preference tests (Kuder, 1952; Cattell and Eber,
1957; Myers, 1962) and distinguishes an interest in ideas and philosophy
on one hand and practicality, scientific, and tangible interests on the other.

The questionnaire complements the TEQ in determining preference for behavioural and group psychotherapeutic treatments.

The DIQ has high test-retest reliability and there is no relationship of scores with sex. There is some evidence that it may be age related but unequivocal evidence of this is lacking. High scores towards an inner direction of interest represent interest in ideas/philosophy. Low scores towards an outer direction of interest represent practical/scientific interests.

Table 2   Mean DIQ scores of various professional and other groups. Data reproduced by kind permission of Caine, Smail, Wijesinghe, and Winter (1982)

Psychiatric social workers	23.26 S.D. 3.93
Clinical psychologists	19.83 S.D. 4.52
Medical students	14.62 S.D. 6.14
Clerks	13.40 S.D. 6.05
Engineering craftsmen	9.92 S.D. 5.82
Psychiatrists	21.21 S.D. 5.37
Therapeutic community nurses	18.38 S.D. 6.42
General nurses	9.50 S.D. 5.48
Psychiatric nurses	12.35 S.D. 5.92
77 Nurses from Napsbury Hospital (training centre of nurses undertaking ENB Course 953)	12.09 S.D. 4.85

Wilson–Patterson Attitude Inventory

The WPAI (Wilson, 1975) is one of the most widely used attitude questionnaires in the world and is essentially an index of conservatism. The author stresses three aspects of the scale: (a) resistance to change,

(b) preference for the traditional, and (c) moderation and cautiousness. The scale has norms for many occupational groups in many different countries. Not surprisingly it is related to age, and females score consistently more conservatively. Higher scores represent higher levels of conservatism.

The Eysenck Personality Questionnaire

The EPQ (Eysenck and Eysenck, 1975) a very widely used measure of personality. It was chosen because the subscales yield three main dimensions of personality, i.e. extroversion, neuroticism and psychoticism, of which established behavioural patterns may be seen as corollaries. Further, it seemed important to establish whether any relationship was apparent between these subscales and the various attitude measures. The questionnaire also obtains a 'Lie' scale which may be simply viewed as measuring the subjects desire to present as socially desirable.

Hypotheses

In view of the fact that the study is a pilot attempt to measure nurses' attitudes to psychiatric/psychological treatment the hypotheses were necessarily rather broad.

Predictions regarding scores on the Attitudes to Treatment Questionnaire

It was predicted that the group of trainee nurse therapists would score (pre-training) lower, i.e. more psychological, less organic, than the other two groups and decrease significantly over training. Also predicted was a statistically significant change (in a lower direction) over training in the group undertaking the Developments in Psychiatric Nursing (ENB 953) course. It was thought that there would be no significant change in the scores of the Nursing Elderly People (ENB 941) course members.

Predictions Concerning the Treatment Expectancy Questionnaire

It was predicted that pre-training the group of trainee nurse therapists would score higher (more behavioural/medical, less towards group psychotherapy) than the other two groups. It was further predicted that the scores of the trainee nurse therapists would change over training to significantly higher scores (more behavioural/medical) while the group undertaking the Developments in Psychiatric Nursing course would change over training to significantly lower scores (more group psychotherapeutic). It was thought that there would be no significant change in the scores of the Nursing Elderly People course members.

Predictions regarding the Direction of Interest Questionnaire

It was predicted that the two groups of psychiatric nurses (courses No. 650 and 953) would score higher (i.e. more inner directed interests) than the Nursing Elderly People Course (No. 941) group before training. No specific predictions regarding differences between the two psychiatric groups were made. It was further predicted that, over training, the nurse therapy group would change to significantly lower (more outer, i.e. practical interest) scores, while the Developments in Psychiatric Nursing would change to significantly higher (more inner, i.e. philosophical) scores. It was predicted that the scores in the Nursing Elderly People group would not significantly change.

Predictions regarding
The Wilson–Patterson Attitude Inventory

It was predicted that the Nursing Elderly group would score higher (more conservative) than the other two groups, pre-treatment, but no specific predictions regarding other differences or changes were made.

Predictions regarding the
Eysenck Personality Questionnaire

No specific predictions regarding scores on this questionnaire were made, as the main object of including this was to establish relationship to attitude measure scores.

Analyses

A parametric analysis was chosen as the scores followed a distribution which approximated to normal. Anderson (1961) has argued authoritatively for the use of parametric analyses with these type of data. Student's independent and related t-tests were used to compute differences between mean scores, within and between subject groups. Pearson's product moment correlation was used to correlate sets of scores. Snodgrass (1980) was used as a reference manual.

Table 3 Mean questionnaire scores (with ages) and related *t*-tests (pre/post-training)

	Age in years	Attitude to Treatment Questionnaire (ATQ)		Treatment Expectancy Questionnaire (TEQ)		Direction of Interest Questionnaire (DIQ)		Wilson–Patterson Attitude Inventory (WPAI)	
		Pre-Training	Post-Training	Pre-Training	Post-Training	Pre-Training	Post-Training	Pre-Training	Post-Training
Nurse Therapy Trainees (ENB 650) n = 8	27.75 S.D. 2.87	41.0 S.D. 8.85	34.80 S.D. 7.99	27.25 S.D. 2.76	24.25 S.D. 3.81	15.00 S.D. 3.85	16.33 S.D. 6.25	23.67 S.D. 12.12	24.17 S.D. 13.48
		$t = 1.93\ p < 0.05$		$t = 2.81\ p < 0.025$		$t = 0.47$ n.s.		$t = 0.76$ n.s.	
Developments in Psychiatric Nursing Course (ENB 953) n = 21	34.81 S.D. 5.84	46.70 S.D. 7.12	43.95 S.D. 6.38	28.61 S.D. 6.99	27.20 S.D. 7.16	14.40 S.D. 7.16	15.00 S.D. 6.85	36.70 S.D. 10.34	36.60 S.D. 10.18
		$t = 1.29$ n.s.		$t = 0.63$ n.s.		$t = 0.27$ n.s.		$t = 0.03$ n.s.	
Nursing Elderly People Course (ENB 941) n = 15	37.73 S.D. 9.68	50.43 S.D. 8.19	49.43 S.D. 11.29	32.00 S.D. 8.98	31.29 S.D. 9.70	10.71 S.D. 4.41	10.57 S.D. 5.40	48.20 S.D. 10.66	47.20 S.D. 10.86
		$t = 0.31$ n.s.		$t = 0.51$ n.s.		$t = 0.12$ n.s.		$t = 0.59$ n.s.	
Trained Nurse Therapists n = 30	33.07 S.D. 4.53	36.37 S.D. 7.59				15.40 S.D. 6.83			

Significance levels for one tailed tests

Results

Results are detailed in Tables 3, 4, 5, 6, and 7.

Regarding the specific hypotheses, the trainee nurse therapist group (ENB 650) scored significantly lower on the ATQ (more psychological, less organic) than the other two groups pre-training. The Developments in Psychiatric Nursing (ENB 953) group mean ATQ score, pre-training, was less than the Nursing Elderly People (ENB 941) group, but this did not reach significance. Only the ENB 650 group changed significantly on this measure.

Contrary to prediction, there was no statistical significance in TEQ scores pre-training, and contrary to expectation the ENB 650 group scored lower (significant $p < 0.025$) post-training. This represents a change to the

Table 4   Mean Eysenck Personality Questionnaire scale scores for experimental groups and from validation data

	L Scale	N Scale	P Scale	E Scale
Nurse therapy trainees (ENB 650) $n = 8$	2.33 S.D. 0.82	11.67 S.D. 6.83	7.33 S.D. 3.33	13.83 S.D. 5.78
Developments in Psychiatric Nursing Course (ENB 953) $n = 21$	6.05 S.D. 3.27	7.35 S.D. 5.57	4.30 S.D. 2.92	14.75 S.D. 3.67
Nursing Elderly People Course (ENB 941) $n = 15$	10.14 S.D. 4.31	9.29 S.D. 4.91	3.28 S.D. 2.16	11.14 S.D. 4.97
*General nurses from validation sample	8.00	9.72	3.47	12.93
*Mean for general population (age 30–39)	8.18	10.95	2.73	12.41

*Male and female scores averaged

Table 5 Comparison between the groups on all pre-treatment measures using independent t-tests

Measure	Nurse Therapy Trainees (ENB 650) versus Developments in Psychiatric Nursing (ENB 953)			Developments in Psychiatric Nursing (ENB 953) versus Nursing Elderly People (ENB 941)			Nurse Therapy Trainees (ENB 650) versus Nursing Elderly People (ENB 941)		
	t	p	d.f.	t	p	d.f.	t	p	d.f.
ATQ*	1.79	<0.05	26	1.45	n.s.	33	2.61	<0.01	21
WP*	2.87	<0.005	26	3.21	<0.005	33	5.01	<0.0005	21
DIQ*	0.22	n.s.	26	1.79	<0.05	33	2.39	<0.025	21
TEQ*	0.53	n.s.	26	1.36	n.s.	33	1.55	n.s.	21
AGE	3.39	<0.005	26	1.01	n.s.	33			
L-scale† (EPQ)	2.98	<0.01	26	3.13	<0.01	33	5.14	<0.0005	21
N-scale† (EPQ)	1.76	n.s.	26	1.11	n.s.	33	0.96	n.s.	21
P-scale† (EPQ)	2.44	<0.05	26	1.08	n.s.	33	3.79	<0.002	21
E-scale† (EPQ)	0.39	n.s.	26	2.48	<0.02	33	1.14	n.s.	21

*Significance level for one-tailed test.
†Significance level for two-tailed test.

more group psychotherapeutic end of the TEQ rather than the medical/behavioural. Contrary to prediction, there was no significant change in the ENB 953 group.

Regarding the DIQ scores, the two psychiatric groups ENB 650 and ENB 953 differed significantly from the ENB 941 group as per prediction (i.e. more inner directed scores) but contrary to prediction neither group changed significantly over training.

On the Wilson–Patterson Inventory (WPAI) the ENB 941 group scored significantly higher (more conservative) than the two psychiatric groups and the ENB 953 group scored significantly higher (more conservative) than the ENB 650 group. None of the groups changed significantly over training.

A comparison of scores of the experimental groups (Table 3) with the scores of various professional groups raises some interesting points. On the ATQ all three groups score lower than comparable professional groups. For example, the ENB 941 course score 11.29 less than a group of General Hospital nurses. Likewise, the ENB 953 course score 6.74 lower than a group of 77 nurses from the hospital in which the course is run. The trainee nurse therapist group score much lower than other psychiatric nurse groups, and at post-training achieve scores of the same order as a group of staff from therapeutic communities.

The comparison of DIQ scores yields less dramatic results although both psychiatric groups (ENB 953 and 650) score higher (more inner directed) than comparable groups of psychiatric nurses.

The EPQ scores (Table 4) reveal dramatic differences on the L scale (large significant differences between all groups) and the mean scores and independent t-tests (Table 5) show that on all comparisons of the groups there are two or more differences between the four scales.

Table 6   Correlations with the Attitudes to Treatment Questionnaire (ATQ)

	ATQ		Change in ATQ	
	r	p	r	p
L-scale (of EPQ)	0.451	<0.01		
Age	0.555	<0.001	0.148	n.s.
Conservatism (Wilson–Patterson)	0.618	<0.001		

Significance levels for two-tailed tests.

Table 7 Comparison of trained nurse therapists

Group	Age	Group difference	ATQ score	Group difference	DIQ score	Group difference
Trained Nurse Therapists n = 30	33.07 S.D. 4.53	t = 3.13	34.80 S.D. 7.99	t = 0.405 n.s.	15.40 S.D. 6.83	t = 0.391 n.s.
Trainee Nurse Therapists n = 8	27.75 S.D. 2.87	p < 0.005	36.37 S.D. 7.59		16.33 S.D. 6.25	
Correlation of ATQ score with time since completing ENB 650 n = 30			0.101 n.s.			

Time since training:
mean = 3.3 years
S.D. = 2.12 range 1–9 years

The ATQ scores were correlated with the L scale of the EPQ, the Wilson–Patterson (conservatism) scale, and age. All three correlations were highly significant (Table 6). A correlation between change in ATQ scores and age did not reach significance.

The trainee nurse therapist's scores on the DIQ and ATQ post-training did not differ significantly from the scores of a group of 30 nurse therapists who had completed ENB course 650. Their range of post-ENB experience (1 to 9 years) did not correlate with ATQ scores.

Discussion

The results of this pilot study raise some interesting issues and certainly indicate future research. On the five measures of change, the groups differ quite considerably. A general description of the groups on the basis of these measures seems worthwhile.

The trainee nurse therapists are the least conservative of the groups and on this measure differ considerably from most psychiatric nurses. On the treatment questionnaires (the ATQ and TEQ) they give responses of a similar nature to staff working within liberal regimes such as therapeutic communities and again differ significantly from the other two experimental groups. In general terms the trainee nurse therapists would favour treatment programmes where the emphasis was on a personal approach, away from hard and fast rules and autocratic treatment ideology. Regarding treatment preferences using the TEQ, their scores are certainly away from the organic and towards 'group psychotherapeutic'. There is also evidence from the reference group data that the experimental group after training are no different in these respects to trained nurse therapists, and there is further evidence from the ATQ and DIQ scores that these attitudes remain over post-training experience. The significant change in questionnaire score over training also give some indicators of the training centre. The broad change to a more 'psychological' personal approach to people and their problems is congruent with the basic philosophy of nurse therapy training where the emphasis is on detailed individual assessment and the tailormaking of behavioural programmes to take into account the unique nature of each patient, drawing from aspects of their social circumstances, relationships, belief, and philosophical views. Of paramount importance in training would be the emphasis on the process of therapist-patient mutual negotiation during all phases of assessment and treatment. Such practices would be at variance with the view of the ATQ and TEQ authors, Caine et al. (1981), who say that behaviour therapy at times amounts to no more than symptom removal by a narrow range of techniques used in cookbook fashion. In drawing up the scales, this view seemed to be the factor in putting behavioural regimes alongside organic and impersonal approaches to patient care. Further, their study of treatment outcome seemed to represent only a narrow group of procedures currently used with neurotic patients, with many references to systematic desensitization as a core treatment. This mode of treatment is not commonly used and is viewed by many as an anachronism. The data from the current study would indicate that the current practice of behaviour therapy may well be very different from that found in their research and that their description of the 'Personal Style' of the therapist carrying out behavioural procedures may be out of date.

With regard to the nurses undertaking the developments in psychiatric nursing course, their questionnaire profile indicates that they too differ from psychiatric nurses in general, although such differences are of a much smaller order than the nurse therapy trainees. This difference may well be demonstrating that such courses preach to the converted, or at least open minded, in that applications for this course may well be coming from a more enlightened group who wish such further training. This, of course, will become an important issue if mandatory refresher courses are instituted. Even so the changes that occur over training are small. This may be that 29 days of exposure to new ideas may be insufficient. This would agree with Hall's (1974) finding, but an alternative explanation would be that a somewhat already enlightened group have reached a ceiling point. The pilot data certainly give no impression that such enlightenment is restricted to the younger nurses in the study. This is verified by the lack of correlation between change in ATQ and Age and by examination of individual cases.

The scores of the control group i.e. Nursing Elderly People course members indicate again that, although they are the most conservative, traditionally minded group, their scores on the various scales show that their overall attitudes regarding psychological treatment are more liberal than their general hospital colleagues. The lack of change over training was predicted, but of interest is an examination of individual cases showing a large variation and, in effect, a cancelling out of changes, because of scores changing in both directions. This could be an issue of questionnaire response, but this is unlikely, if one takes into account the test-retest reliability of all but one of the scales. The issue of individual response is clearly important and can only be investigated adequately using a multifaceted evaluation procedure.

Regarding the EPQ scale, it seems clear that the three groups are very different. There are highly significant differences on the L-scale between the groups, and other significant differences of the P- and N-scale. Eysenck and Eysenck (1975) do suggest some procedures for correcting dependent variables when certain scale patterns become apparent, but the number of subjects in this study is too small to consider such a procedure.

The scores on the main measure of attitude (the ATQ) in this study are correlated very highly with age, L-scale, and conservatism. The latter correlation was described in the source book but was of a lower order (0.50 as opposed to 0.618). The L-scale finding is the most interesting.

The L-scale can be viewed as a validity check for respondents giving answers which they see as socially acceptable rather than what they really believe. The ATQ scale has no such inbuilt device and the study finding indicates that this matter should be further investigated. Certainly this finding indicates that attitude research in the nurse education area should take into account the issue of giving socially acceptable answers.

Generally the results of the pilot study indicate that evaluation of attitudes to treatment or courses designed to influence nurses attitudes should incorporate other measures. Milne (1984) used a procedure incorporating skill and learning measures including a procedure similar to the 'critical incident' technique (Ryback, 1967). His measures seemed to be sensitive to training effects but lacked an *in vivo* component. Ideally one would wish to follow up nurses into their clinical environment. Brooker and Wiggins (1983) did just that but their research was retrospective and lacked systematic evaluation of attitude variables.

This study has provided the ground work for future evaluation of nurse training courses which should incorporate multiple measures of change together with the measurement of the behavioural sequelae of training.

Summary

The literature concerning attitudes to treatment and in particular nurses' attitudes is reviewed. The study investigated changes in attitude over training using five measures. Three groups of nurses were evaluated pre- and post-training. These groups were trainee nurse therapists (ENB Course 650), Nurses Undertaking Developments in Psychiatric Nursing (ENB 953) and nurses undertaking the course Nursing Elderly People (ENB 941). A fourth reference group of trained nurse therapists was assessed and used for comparative purposes.

The results indicated that all three groups differed considerably in their attitude to psychological treatment and on personality variables. Nurse therapist trainees changed the most and perhaps surprisingly towards a preference for more liberal regimes. Some questions regarding the Attitudes to Treatment Questionnaire have been raised by the study. The current study has indicated the need for larger scale research using more general measurement including direct behavioural observation.

Acknowledgments

My grateful thanks to Miss Brenda Shelton, Mrs Erica Jacyna, and Mr Erville Millar (course tutors for ENB courses 941, 953, and 650, respectively) for their cooperation, Dr David Winter of Napsbury Hospital for his support during the project and advice on the data relating to the Claybury Battery, and Mrs Jean Gournay for help with the statistical analysis.

References

Ajzen, I. and Fishbein, M. (1980). *Understanding Attitudes and Predicting Social Behaviour*. Prentice-Hall. Englewood Cliffs, New Jersey.

Anderson, N. H. (1961). Scales and Statistics: Parametric and Non-parametric. *Psychological Bulletin*, **58** (4), 305–316.

Brooker, C. and Wiggins, R.D. (1983). Nurse-therapist trainee variability: The implications for selection and training. *Journal of Advanced Nursing*, **8**, 321–328.

Caine, T. M. and Smail, D. J. (1968). Attitudes of psychiatric nurses to their role in treatment. *British Journal of Medical Psychology*, **41**, 193–197.

Caine, T. M., Wijesinghe, O. B. A., and Winter, D. A. (1981). *Personal Styles in Neurosis: Implications for Small Group Psychotherapy and Behaviour Therapy*. Routledge and Kegan Paul, London.

Caine, T. M., Smail, D. J., Wijesinghe, O. B. A., and Winter, D. A. (1982). *The Claybury Selection Battery Manual*. NFER-Nelson, Windsor.

Cattell, R. B. and Eber, H. W. (1957). *Handbook for the Sixteen Personality Factor Questionnaire*. Institute of Personality and Ability testing, Illinois.

Eysenck, H. J. and Eysenck, S. B. G. (1975). *The Manual of the Eysenck Personality Questionnaire* Hodder and Stoughton, Sevenoaks.

Hall, J. N. (1974). Nurse attitudes and specialized treatment settings. An exploratory study. *British Journal of Social and Clinical Psychology*, **13**, 333–334.

Jones, R. G. and Galliard, P. G. (1983). Exploratory study to evaluate staff attitudes towards geriatric psychiatry. *Journal of Advanced Nursing*, **8**, 47–57.

Kuder, G. F. (1952). *The Kuder Preference Record (Personal Form A. H.)*. Science Research Associates, Chicago, USA.

Lillie, F. J. (1973). Psychiatry and mental distress, in Wilson G. D. (Ed.), *The Psychology of Conservatism*. Academic Press, London.

Krech, D. and Crutchfield, R. S. (1948). *Theory and Problems in Social Psychology*. McGraw-Hill, New York.

Marks, I. M., Hallam, R. S., Connolly, J., and Philpott, R. (1977). *Nursing in Behaviour Psychotherapy*. RCN Publications, London.

Milne, D. (1984). The relevance of nurses' characteristics in learning behaviour therapy. *Journal of Advanced Nursing*, **9**, 175–179.

Myers, I. B. (1962). *Manual for the Myers-Briggs Type Indicator Educational Testing Service.* Princeton, USA.

O'Leary, K. D. (1984). The image of behaviour therapy: It is time to take a stand. *Behaviour Therapy*, **15** (3), 219–233.

Rosenberg, M. J. and Hovland, C. I. (1960). Cognitive, affective and behavioural components of attitudes, in Hovland, C. I. and Rosenberg, M. J. (Eds), *Attitude Organization and Change.* Yale University Press, New Haven, Connecticut. Connecticut.

Ryback, D. (1967). A critical incident simulation technique for nurse selection. *International Journal of Nursing Studies*, **4**, 81–89.

Shanley, E. (1981). Attitudes of Psychiatric Hospital Staff towards mental illness. *Journal of Advanced Nursing*, **6**, 199–203.

Snodgrass, J. N. (1980). *The Numbers Game: Statistics for Psychology.* Oxford University Press, New York.

Trauer, T. (1977). Attitudes of psychiatric patients to staff roles and treatment methods: A replication and extension. *British Journal of Medical Psychology*, **50**, 39–44.

Wilson, G. D. (1975). The Wilson–Patterson Attitude Inventory (WPAI). NFER Publishing, Windsor.

Winter, D. A., Brown, R. J., Roitt, M., Shivakumar, H., Jones, S., Connoly, D. J., Acton, T., Arzoumawides, J., and Beeson, S. (1985). Evaluation of a crisis intervention service. 1. Staff attitudes. *British Journal of Psychiatry* (submitted for publication).

CHAPTER 5

The Strain of Training:
Being a Student
Psychiatric Nurse

BRYN DAVIS

Editor's Comments

Bryn Davis provides valuable insights into student nurse socialization. He
used semi-structured interviews and Repertory Grid technique to obtain
descriptive data about student psychiatric nurses, their perceptions of
nursing and of themselves, and their problems in adjusting to psychiatric
nursing. On the basis of his findings Bryn Davis advocates that students'
progress through the stressful process of becoming psychiatric nurses
should be monitored, to facilitate coping strategies and permit helpful
interventions to take place.

'I just burst into tears—I didn't like it at all!'
(2nd year student psychiatric nurse)

Introduction

Many student nurses experience problems and stress during training.
Problems of course may not be insurmountable and, indeed, the process
of training is to enable the student to learn how to deal with them. If the
student copes with the problem, she meets a challenge, and this gives her
the satisfaction that is often its own reward. However, if the nurse cannot
cope, she experiences stress and, all too frequently, is unable to complete
her training. It seems that the first year of training is the most stressful,
and that the highest proportion of learners who give up their training do
so within the first six months (Macguire, 1969; Birch, 1975). This applies

to all branches of nursing, but particularly to psychiatric nurse training (Davis, 1983a). Although there has been much research into the selection and recruitment of nurse trainees (Lewis, 1983), relatively little exists into the perceptions and reactions of students undergoing psychiatric nurse training, e.g. Towell (1975). Recently, however, there have been other developments in this area, e.g. Powell (1982) and Clinton (1981). The process of student nurse socialization is just beginning to get the attention it needs.

What is meant by this term 'socialization'? One definition is that it is the process by which individuals acquire the knowledge, skills, and dispositions that enable them to participate as more or less effective members of groups, organizations or society itself (Brim, 1966). This involves changes in the nature and integration of the social selves from which the individual selects that one most suited to a particular setting. This self is developed in relation to experiences of that setting and is not predictable from a knowledge of personality or intellectual factors (Schein, 1971).

This picture gives us a view of adult socialization as involving the creation of a social self related to the perceived expectations of a particular aspect of the world, role, social setting being entered by the trainee. An active role is played by the recruit, but the organization usually offers support to the process, that is significant others, who help. From the extensive literature on the subject, five main factors can be identified:

anticipatory socialization;
stress experiences;
peer group support;
perceptions of significant others;
development of the self (Davis, 1983a).

Adult reference groups and significant others are influential in supporting decisions to enter training. Peer group support is invaluable in coming to terms with the conflict between expectations and experiences, and in finding out what the job is about. Significant others, during training, offer and may provide support or act as models for the trainee, and the self concept is enlarged to incorporate the new social self being developed, in this case student nurse and nurse. Student nurse training has much in common with preparation for entry to other professions, such as medicine, the church, and officer status in the armed forces. Here the main influence is from a tradition of hallowed leaders, and from intellectual and cultural aspects supporting the academic part of training. However, nurse training also has much in common with entry to other occupations, such as the police, and other ranks in the armed forces. Influences in these settings come from strict processes and procedures devised to reduce individuality. These involve institutional living accommodation, uniforms, hair styles, and other aspects of appearance, total devotion to duty, availability for unsocial hours of duty, and unpleasant work subject to pressures of time and accuracy. Punishments can be brutal, emotionally if not physically.

The picture, recently, in nurse training is changing, and particularly with regard to psychiatric nurse training, where much more relaxed attitudes frequently exist. Nevertheless, the process of student nurse socialization is one that involves a unique mixture of influences and processes that warrant serious study. This chapter consists of three sections. The first section shows the reactions of a sample of eight and five student psychiatric nurses in two schools of nursing to their training. These are derived from a series of semi-structured interviews at the end of the first year. The next section is concerned with an attempt to study more systematically student nurses' perceptions of their training. In particular this section considers what kind of people the students were, and how they saw themselves during the first year of training. The third and final part consists of a discussion of the implications of the two preceding sections.

Reactions to Psychiatric Nurse Training

'I remember being absolutely terrified',
'I felt homesick and sad',
'The actual ward experience I find most rewarding'.
(2nd year student psychiatric nurses)

These are verbatim comments by student psychiatric nurses at the end of their first year of training. They are taken from a series of interviews with students undergoing two types of training, general and psychiatric. The study, and the results from the two groups, unseparated, have been reported elsewhere (Davis 1984). Here it is proposed to concentrate on the findings relating to the student psychiatric nurses. Comments by the students were obtained in semi-structured interviews about a range of topics. These statements were then categorized into themes in association with the students during group discussions. Four of these main themes will be described in the students' own words, the relative importance of the themes being assessed by the amount of comment they generated.

The First Day on the Ward

The major theme causing most comment was that of the students' remembered emotional reactions to their first day on the ward. The comments quoted at the beginning of this section belong to this theme. Twice as many negative comments were made as positive. Other negative comments included:

'You felt so lost',
'I was apprehensive',
'I didn't expect it to be like that'.

These statements certainly highlight the importance of this first experience for the students, and the stress that can be associated with it. Some students, however, felt the opposite, as the following positive statements show:

'I felt most confident and relaxed',
'I felt at home, more bustle, more variety'.

The ward experience, described in such different ways, occurred after introductory blocks where the students were introduced to the concepts involved in mental health and illness, and also to some of the practicalities of caring for the mentally ill. Also included had been short visits to the wards for illustrative and practice sessions. Nevertheless, these reactions occurred when the students were allocated to their first full-time ward experience.

Kramer (1974) has described similar reactions as 'reality shock', when reported in studies of student nurse socialization in America. The reality of nursing after all the anticipations and perhaps the more idealized view obtained from the school of nursing, can provide a contrast that is very difficult to cope with. Other studies in America have reported emotional reactions to ward experience too (e.g. Olesen and Whittaker, 1968). However, these have been concerned with general students. In the UK similar findings have also been reported (e.g. Melia, 1983; Davis, 1984). As mentioned in the Introduction, reports of the experiences of student psychiatric nurses have not been so forthcoming, but some information is available in Towell (1975), Powell (1982), and Clinton (1981). The reactions described here echo those in these American and British studies and seem to relate to an important aspect of socialization: that of crossing the boundary into the world of nursing and the role of nurse. This psychological adjustment can be anticipated and prepared for, and is the purpose of the introductory period. However, stress is still frequently experienced. Support, from peer group, from models, from tutors, if not present can raise the height of the psychological barrier to be crossed.

Nurse training is essentially an apprenticeship and the new recruit becomes a nurse by doing nursing with the rest of the health care team. It can be, and is, argued that students must learn to cope for themselves; not to be too dependent and so on. The kind of nurses they become depends on their initiative, knowledge gained from books and lectures, and, perhaps most important, from others in the clinical setting. The problem seems to be that all too frequently the students are on their own without suitable support, guidance, and example from experienced staff.

Support and Guidance

The comments made by the student psychiatric nurses about the nature of the support and guidance that they felt they did receive were evenly divided into positive and negative, and form the next major theme in the analysis. A key comment was: 'I prefer to ask someone who's not going to bite my head off'. This emphasizes also the importance of personality and interpersonal relationships in the process of becoming a professional. This involves social skills on the part of the teacher or charge nurse or other significant person, as well as their availability and accessibility. The following statements illustrate the kind of relationships seen as important and supportive by the students.

'The charge nurse kept me under his wing for the first 48 hours, until I knew the routine',
'We all worked together',
'Anything you want to know, you can ask',

They compare with such statements as:

'I got no guidance whatsoever',
'I was usually on my own',
'Charge nurse says, "I'm busy, come back later"'.

Considering these different kinds of reaction, and that the sample came from two different psychiatric hospitals, the question of how the students knew what the job was about on the ward can be posed. This was the next major theme arising from the students' comments.

Knowing what the Job is about

Half of the comments were directed at being prepared, and the remainder at being left to find out for themselves. Examples of the former are:

'You get the basic facts in school, and on the ward you see it in reality',
'It's when you go on the ward, after the school that it fits',
'I learn most by doing'.

These latter comments seem to be related to those reflecting a positive reaction to the ward experiences and emphasize the importance of clinical experience in the process of becoming a nurse. It is in coping with these stresses and challenges on the ward that the socialization process occurs. The negative comments concerning knowing what the job is about on the ward reflect a lack of preparation and a strain on the commitment and initiative of the students:

'I didn't understand what I was supposed to do',
'It was left up to us to find our own way',
'I learnt by trial and error'.

That so many do succeed in becoming qualified nurses confirms their commitment and initiative. However, it seems an expensive, wasteful way to train nurses, allowing them, in this unsupported, unprepared way to create psychiatric nursing afresh for themselves, or to pick up knowledge and practices from other than the nurse teaching team. Other evidence indicates that nursing auxiliaries, non-nursing friends, and parents are frequently used as resources (Davis 1983a).

Similar results to these have been reported for general student nurses. For example, Melia (1983) describes it as 'working in the dark'. The variety of responses, however, indicates that some students were receiving and appreciating help in crossing the boundary into the nursing role, and in playing that role. The kind of nurses that they become is going to be influenced by their guides and mentors. Those who do not receive this support become 'nurses' without this influence, using their own, and perhaps their peer group's initiative. This is one way to achieve innovation in nursing. Whether it is the best or even a desirable way is not clear.

The stresses associated with the first few days of experience on a new ward or in a different clinical situation can so easily be reduced by a supportive role from the senior experienced nurses. This guides the learner into the practices, knowledge, and attitudes to be acquired during that experience. If occurring when needed, such support soon strengthens the student to be more effective and independent.

Interpersonal Relationships

A few statements highlighted in particular the theme of interpersonal relationships, showing that because they developed, coping was possible:

'I was fortunate to have a friend there',
'It's much easier to work in a relaxed atmosphere',
'It was hard work, but you need cooperation from staff'.

Not only is socialization into nursing dependent on experience, under the supervision and modelling of teachers and senior nurses, but job satisfaction seems to be directly associated with caring for patients, as far as the student psychiatric nurses were concerned:

'I like doing things for patients',
'I like being appreciated by patients',
'I like talking to patients — working with people',
'I like seeing an improvement in patients'.

It is possible of course that what gives the learners the most satisfaction is not 'good nursing' or not relevant to their curriculum of experience. Nevertheless, it is important for the nurse educators to be aware of the learners' own needs. When planning a teaching curriculum and a programme of experience together with the associated tutorial support, the active role played by the student must be considered. If not, the active role may conflict with the prescribed role, to the detriment not only of the student's training, but also to the care that is given. Student nurses, like any other people in social settings, act, react, and interact. Becoming a nurse is a process, shared by the student, her significant others from whom she accepts advice and guidance and to whom she turns for support and friendship, and the clinical setting in which the experience is gained. All too frequently nurse educators are imposing a training scheme, rather than sharing in this process. A sensitivity to the student's reactions would indicate such participation.

Profiles of the Student Psychiatric Nurses

In this section findings from a more systematic study of student psychiatric nurses are presented and discussed. The project and method used have

Table 1   Results from the Personal Questionnaire comparing 22 student psychiatric
nurses with 17 general student nurses

Characteristic	Psychiatric student nurses ($n = 22$)	General student nurses ($n = 17$)
Age on leaving school	16 years 10 months	16 years 11 months
Age on entry to training	25 years 2 months	19 years 8 months*
Qualifications on entry		
GNC	25%	
'O' level/CSE/GNC	50%	80%
'A' level	25%	20%
Previous nursing experience		
student	5%	6.25%
cadet	–	25%*
Previous work experience	90%	75%
Residence		
Nurses Home	55%	81.25%
Spouse	20%	12.5%*
Parents	15%	6.25%
Flat	10%	–

*Statistically significant difference, $\alpha = p < 0.05$.

been described elsewhere (Davis, 1983b). Briefly, twenty-two students were asked to describe themselves, others in their professional settings, and their family and friends using a specially developed Repertory Grid, (Kelly, 1955; Fransella and Bannister, 1977). The descriptions were created from comparisons between the various individuals involved, so that two were seen as alike and different from one other, by the student. From the ways in which the students saw themselves and their significant others as being alike or different, the profiles were produced. The students were also asked to complete a personal questionnaire, the results of which are now presented.

Characteristics

As illustrated in Table 1, the student psychiatric nurses differed in certain ways from general student nurses. They were on average significantly older; fewer had previous nursing experience although a majority had previous

Table 2   List of categories used in the analysis of
constructs elicited from the student psychiatric nurses

Categories	Explanation
Personal/psychological	Attributes (behavioural or psychological) of a general or personal nature
Role	Attributes of a professional nature or relating to the work situation
Interaction	Involving being in contact with or working with
Communication	Involving talking or confiding
Self-image	Attributes, behaviour or situations involving self
Authority	Attributes expressing positions in a hierarchy, or being in charge or in control

working experience; and far more lived out of the hospital with a spouse, parents or in a flat. Although of interest in themselves, these results also have relevance to the interpretation of the findings which follow.

Professional Self-image

The words used to describe the student nurses and their significant others were categorized in order to study further various aspects of self in relation to others and, in particular, the developing professional self-image of the students themselves. The results applying to student psychiatric nurses are presented and discussed here. The categories into which the descriptions (constructs) were placed are shown in Table 2.

At the beginning of training, the student psychiatric nurses saw themselves, in terms of role, as being:

'Involved in the needs of the ward',
'Concerned with practice'

and as

'wanting to learn'.

When asked to make the same comparisons and descriptions after nine months training, they saw themselves as being;

'Taught in school and on the wards',
'Still in training',
'Successfully trained to help patients'.

Thus the students have a strong perception of self as learners, which, at nine months, is showing some signs of becoming nurses, as well as being involved in the practical ward work. This strong self-image is confirmed by constructs in the category self-image at the beginning of training;

'Desire to be successful in dealing with patients',
'I want to be a student nurse',
'Identify with other nurses'.

The following constructs are from nine months later;

'I want to be what I am',
'The present and future me'.

This is a picture of confidence and assertion, of knowing who one is and where one is going. Further evidence to support this comes from the personal, psychological attributes which were classed in the category 'Personal' at the beginning of training;

'Active',
'Confident',
'Close association',

and from nine months later:

'No frills',
'Reality (the real thing)',
'Still achieving'.

The student psychiatric nurses were very much involved with the ward work, as shown above, and saw themselves as having close associations with their colleagues, illustrated by such constructs as:

'Work together on the wards',
'Helping together'.

Some evidence from studies utilizing personality tests and attitude scales indicates that recruits to nursing tend to be psychologically vulnerable people (Davis, 1983a), and this was reflected in some of the comments quoted in the first section, from the interviews with student psychiatric nurses about their early experiences. However, there is also evidence of a strong commitment often maintained over long periods prior to entry to training. There is also evidence that student psychiatric nurses experience periods of confusion and uncertainty, particularly with respect to the resource people available for help with problems anticipated or encountered. (Davis, 1983b). Self has also been shown to be a major resource. This strong sense of self perhaps reflects the greater maturity (in terms of age at least) of these students. Also linked with this self-confident image may be the fact that they tend not to live in the nurses' home and have had to cope as individuals in other work settings.

General Self-image

When asked to compare themselves with family and friends, as well as with mental health care professionals, a more general picture emerges of the student psychiatric nurses. They claimed to know themselves well, to be responsible and efficient, and to have had this awareness of self for a long time. This again reflects their sense of maturity, even at the beginning of training. Later at nine months, they stated themselves to be good company, young, nice and kind, but suffering from confusion. This latter attribute shows perhaps their desire to be a nurse and yet their awareness of their strong links with non-professionals (family and friends) and their own state of not yet being trained.

When the constructs categorized under Professional are considered further, we see evidence to support this interpretation:

'Unqualified',
'Non-professional',
'a student',
'training to be a nurse'.

These constructs were applied to self at the end of the first nine months of training. We thus have a quite complex and sophisticated picture of the self-image of student psychiatric nurses, both from the interviews presented in the first section and from the images of self from the Repertory Grid Study. In the final section the implications of this picture are discussed and some suggestions made for the utilization of such findings.

Implications

With any research project, the results are always subject to the question of how far we can generalize from them to other situations. This is in many ways an irrelevant question, when the specific findings from a small scale study involve a convenience sample, as reported here. These results, of course, must be situation specific in terms of the constructs elicited and the changes and developments demonstrated. What can be generalized, however, are the principles, or the processes highlighted by these findings. Much research in the social sciences attempts to emulate the physical sciences, in finding or proposing general laws of behaviour which will apply on all occasions and in all situations. Yet, most interpersonal, social situations are relatively unique, in the mix of people involved, the organizational and structural aspects of the setting, and the goals or objectives. Because of this dynamic, fluid state, behaviour is most difficult to predict. However, it can be more easily understood, afterwards, in the light of various very general laws.

Consequently, when trying to predict the outcome of a training programme, given a particular set of recruits, teachers, models, and experiences, we as a profession can appear to be relatively inefficient, and wastage rates or failure rates can reach alarming proportions. Attempts to decide which potential recruits will make successful students or, even more difficult to predict, which will become successful nurses, seem to be doomed to failure. However, rather than prediction, it might be better to monitor the ongoing situation, the process of becoming a nurse. By so doing remedial or adjusting interventions can be made which will ensure that the process pursues its desired course. This assumes, of course, that the desired course is known, and can be achieved. This procedure echoes that for the process of nursing and the monitoring of care plans. Assessment of learner needs, and the implementation of a curriculum to meet those is a distinct parallel. Monitoring evaluations are vital to both settings.

There is now a substantial body of knowledge about the process of becoming a general nurse, and many of the principles from that work can find echoes in psychiatric nursing. In the United States of America, the work of Olesen and Whittaker (1968), Simpson et al. (1979), and Kramer (1974) has contributed much to our understanding. In this country, Melia (1983) and Davis (1983a) have also contributed to this area of knowledge, and have plotted the dimensions of the student nurse's world.

As has been indicated above, nurse training involves a most dynamic social milieu. Tutors are active in planning the academic and experiential aspects of the course as well as providing the former. The clincial staff are active in delivering the care in which the patients also actively participate.

The student psychiatric nurses are not passive in all this, but actively respond to the teaching and to the clinical experience, and make their own contributions. In many instances, as was shown in their own words, they are left alone, to make what they can of the experience. Their emotional reactions to all this can be quite extreme, and result in distress, failure, or rejection of the training. By recognizing the dynamic nature of such social situations, it is possible to institute monitoring or evaluative services which will demonstrate the processes involved at individual or group level, and allow adjustment to be made. The nature of such interventions must depend on the particular problems or discrepancies revealed.

The findings reported here concerning the distress of student psychiatric nurses, their perceptions of self as learners, their relative independence, and their confusion are valuable to those involved in their training. These insights into their views of their experiences and their relationships with others can greatly facilitate the role of tutors in planning the next phases of the course, or the kind of support and guidance that may be most fruitful. This means, as well, that those doing the monitoring and planning the adjustments necessary must have the power and authority to do so.

Much has been said over the last decade or so, of the need for full student status in nurse training. There are strong arguments for and against this development. However, an even stronger argument is beginning to be mounted for the consideration of the active role played by student nurses in their training, whether as 'students' or as 'apprentices'. The processes involved must be assessed, planned for, and evaluated. It is the implementation of an 'educational process' that is being argued here, rather than student status. The 'process' applies to students or apprentices, and side-steps the issue. Concentration on the process involved will give the 'learner' (student or apprentice) the 'status' needed in order to become, in this instance, a psychiatric nurse.

Regular monitoring is a vital part of any process, and techniques are being recognized and developed for this purpose. The method used in the study reported here, of structured interviews using the repertory grid technique, is most adept at eliciting individual learners' accounts of particular situations or problems. It is a format which allows comparisons to be made between assessments so that change or development can be demonstrated. Also, in its method, it provides a useful way of achieving an interactive relationship between the student and the picture revealed. Thus, the individual creating the assessment of the situation, can then indicate, with guidance perhaps, in which way change would be preferable or possible. Alternatively, help can be requested, guidance can be obtained, and new ways of dealing with the situation or problems can be explored, in a systematic, controlled way (Davis 1985).

In this chapter, the comments of a relatively small group of student psychiatric nurses about their experiences and about themselves have been presented and discussed. The students were shown to be relatively independent, aware of their student, 'becoming', status and yet, in the early stages of training, vulnerable to the stresses and strains of their experiences and in need of support and guidance. Coping with stress is, of course, an important part of any achievement, and is rightly part of the process of becoming a psychiatric nurse. However, the emphasis must be on 'coping'. Efficient monitoring of the learners' progress through these experiences and stresses of the course must become an important part of it, if the principles of the present and related research findings are to become part of our body of professional knowledge.

Acknowledgment

The research described in this chapter was undertaken with the support of a DHSS Nursing Research Fellowship.

References

Birch, J. A. (1975). *To Nurse or Not to Nurse*. Royal College of Nursing, London.
Brim, O. G. (1966). Socialisation through the life cycle, in O. G. Brim and S. Wheeler (Eds), *Socialisation after Childhood*. Wiley, New York.
Clinton, M. E. (1981). Training for psychiatric nurses; a sociological study of the problem of integrating theory and practice. PhD Thesis, University of East Anglia, School of Economics and Social Studies.
Davis, B. D. (1983a). A repertory grid study of formal and informal aspects of student nurse training. Unpublished PhD thesis, University of London.
Davis, B. D. (Ed.) (1983b). *Research into Nurse Education*. Croom Helm, Beckenham, Kent.
Davis, B. D. (1984). Interviews with student nurses about their training. *Nurse Education Today*, **4** (6) 136–140.
Davis, B. D. (1985). Dependency grids: an illustration of their use in an educational setting. In N. Beail (Ed.) *Repertory Grid Technique and Personal Constructs*. Croom Helm, Beckenham, Kent.
Fransella, F. and Bannister, D. (1977). *A manual of Repertory Grid Technique*. Academic Press, London.
Kelly, G. A. (1955). *The Psychology of Personal Constructs, vols 1 and 2*. Norton, New York.
Kramer, M. (1974). *Reality Shock: Why Nurses Leave Nursing*. Mosby, St Louis.
Lewis, B. (1983). Personality and intellectual characteristics of trainee nurses and their assessment, in B. D. Davis (Ed.), *Research into Nurse Education*, Croom Helm, Beckenham, Kent.

MacGuire, J. M. (1969). *Threshold to Nursing*. Occasional Papers on Social Administration, No. 30, Bell, London.

Melia, K. M. (1983). Students' views on nursing; a series of papers. *Nursing Times*, **79**, 20–22.

Olesen, V. L. and Whittaker, E. W. (1968). *The Silent Dialogue*. Jossey-Bass Inc., San Francisco.

Powell, D. (1982). *Learning to Relate*. Royal College of Nursing, London.

Schein, E. H. (1971). The individual, the organisation and the carers; a conceptual scheme. *Journal of Applied Behavioural Science*, **7**, 401–426.

Simpson, I. H., Back, K., Ingles, T., Karckhoff, A., and McKinney, J. C. (1979). *From Student to Nurse: a Longitudinal Study of Socialisation*. Cambridge University Press, Cambridge.

Towell, D. (1975). *Understanding Psychiatric Nursing*. Royal College of Nursing, London.

Part C   Patient Care in Psychiatric Nursing

CHAPTER 6

Treatment of Depressed Women by Nurses in Britain and the USA

VERONA GORDON

Editor's Comments

Verona Gordon has carried out several studies in the USA of nursing interventions to reduce depression in women. This chapter is mainly concerned with the replication carried out in Britain when Verona Gordon was a visiting research fellow at Chelsea College, University of London.

The study evaluated a group intervention for depressed women facilitated by psychiatric nurses. Pre- and post-testing showed that women who attended the group sessions showed a significant decrease in depression and significant increase in self-esteem compared with control subjects who received no treatment. The study is important as it is among the very few British studies which evaluate a therapeutic nursing intervention and it clearly demonstrates the ability of nurses to lead an effective treatment programme.

Verona Gordon's careful and detailed account describes a range of measuring instruments which could be of use in other studies. Her study design with randomized control and experimental groups is unusual in psychiatric nursing research and provides a useful model for future treatment evaluations. The design has several important limitations. It is possible that a leaderless group or a group led by any appropriately trained mental health worker would have been just as effective as the nurse-run group. Nevertheless, the study demonstrates that nurses *can* successfully lead groups, in itself an important finding. There was no long-term follow-up, which raises questions about whether the improvements would be maintained. It would have been interesting to investigate whether the work book written by Verona Gordon and used in the group would have been just as effective used alone.

91

The researcher describes in her chapter the overwhelming response to her call for subjects, which confirmed her view of the magnitude of the problem of depression. These women receive little help from the existing services and represent a huge untapped population who could benefit from the skills of psychiatric nurses.

Introduction

Depression ranks as one of the major health problems of women today. Although prominent researchers Weissman and Klerman (1977) reported that twice as many women are depressed as men around the world, few research studies have been published on the development and utilization of treatment approaches to meet the needs of this population. The widespread growth in the number of American females of all ages suffering from depression is alarming (Guttentag *et al.*, 1980). Depressed women have increased medical costs due to their repeated visits to physicians for psychosomatic complaints, chemical dependency, unnecessary gynaecological surgery, and their high psychiatric hospitalizations. Women seek counselling, however, there have been few convincing research studies on the effectiveness of traditional psychotherapies (Fiske *et al.*, 1970). Due to the rising high cost of health care, treatment approaches in mental health must be efficacious, safe and cost-effective (Parloff, 1980). Accelerating societal change is having an impact on women. The challenges to traditional values, roles, and expectations are a source of concern to women and generate emotional responses. Depression is one such emotional response that has been found to be a significant problem among women. Prevention of depression among this segment of society requires an understanding of women's perceptions of, and concerns about, their life situations. Women have high potential to learn, strong interest in growing, great influence over their families, and much to give others.

The purpose of this chapter is to provide more information about the phenomenon of depression in women and to describe a nurse group intervention designed by the author to alleviate depression in women. Several research studies conducted in the United States will be reported as well as a descriptive account of a replicated study completed in London.

Review of the Literature

Forty million Americans suffered from depression today and two-thirds of these people are women (Hirschfield, 1980). Eminent researchers

(Dohrenwend, 1973; van Keep and Prill, 1975; Tucker, 1977; Notman, 1979) identified stressors occurring in women's daily lives which stem from personal, family, social, and cultural demands upon them. These result in feelings of frustration, inadequacy, and low self-esteem.

Problems facing women as they age in America include marital conflicts (Cherlin, 1981), divorce (Gordon, 1979), loss of attractiveness (Scarf, 1980), conflicts at work (Powell, 1977; Shields, 1980), career disruptions due to husband's job change (Weissman *et al.*, 1973), hysterectomy surgery (Editorial, 1979; Raphael, 1976; Martin *et al.*, 1980), 'empty-nest' syndrome (Bart, 1971; Radloff 1975), menopause (Neugarten *et al.*, 1963), widowhood (Lopata, 1971), declining physical health (Wittenborn and Buhler, 1979), and care of elderly parents (Stevenson, 1977). These factors may result in feelings of loneliness and isolation (Gordon, 1982). (There is concern in America in respect to women's influential role in her family and that she has the longest life expectancy, 78 years vs males 70 years, and earns over half of the nation's income.)

Psychological Explanations

There may be three aetiological explanations for these escalating rates of depression in American women as described by theories of:

1 Lewinsohn's behavioural model,
2 Seligman's learned helplessness model,
3 Beck's cognitive model.

From the behavioural viewpoint depression occurs when a women does not perceive positive reinforcement in her daily life (Lewinsohn *et al.*, 1982). The highest rate of depression in American females occurs between the ages of 25 and 44 years, probably their response to their own high expectations of work, marriage or having children. Belle (1982) found low-income single mothers most vulnerable to depression and that the rate of psychiatric treatment of their children was high. Most women working full-time earn 59 per cent less than male full-time workers for doing the same job (Barrett, 1979). Eighty per cent of all women working in America tend to work in demanding 'service' jobs (factory work, cleaning, clerical, bank tellers, sales) which arc low in pay and prestige (National Commission on Working Women, 1979). Women who are employed find social-financial inequality, sex-role stereotyping, and negative prejudice, which result in reduced self-fulfilment and career options (Clayton *et al.*, 1980; Carmen *et al.*, 1981).

Unemployed, married women consistently report frustration with their roles (Neuberry *et al.*, 1979). Housewives have few sources of gratification

(Thurnher, 1976; Radloff and Rae, 1979): their work is relatively invisible and given little value or prestige. The absence of intimate supportive relationships with husband or children increase the risk of depression (Brown *et al.*, 1975; Miller, 1976). The fact that depression is more common among married, divorced or separated women than men is well documented (Radloff, 1975). Gove (1972) reported that the strain of the marriage role is a causal factor of the higher rate of depression among women. The divorce rate in the United States has increased 96 per cent in the last decade and 50 per cent of all future marriages are predicted to end in divorce (*Los Angeles Times*, 1980). The stress of divorce is felt more by women than by men due to women's lack of money, poor living conditions, and lack of job skills (Maykowsky, 1980). Due to present national economy, there are a growing number of women staying in loveless, empty, and abusive marriages (Kaslow, 1982). Pilisuk and Froland (1978) write that depression in women will continue to increase with the high mobility (extended families living thousands of miles apart), small family size, and high divorce rates.

In studies by Wood and Duffy, (1966), Curlee (1969), and McLachlan *et al.* (1976), the middle-aged married housewife, not working outside her home, was found to be a higher consumer of alcohol in attempting to escape her isolation and loneliness.

Seligman's (1975) theory of learned helplessness exemplifies women's hopeless attitude which results in depression, withdrawal, and lack of motivation. There is growing awareness of the powerlessness of women in our male-dominated society, where women do not perceive that they have control over situations or that their actions bring rewards or recognition (LeDray and Chaignot, 1980; Guttentag *et al.*, 1980; Schaef, 1981). Belle's (1982) work with poor single mothers is powerful documentation of their helplessness fighting an indifferent government system. Studies by Chodoff (1972) and Goldberg (1973) report of depressed women with 'helpless' characteristics, and are supported by Radloff and Monroe (1978), Notman *et al.* (1978), and Kivett (1979).

Miller (1976) states that women have been relegated to nurturing tasks and may be forced to decide between either personal growth or development of an intimate relationship with men. The problem of wife-battering has increasingly been brought to the attention of the American public. Claerhout *et al.* (1982) state that violence occurs in 35–50 per cent of all marital relationships and that in part cultural attitudes explain the occurrence. While men are taught to be aggressive and independent, women often assume dependent and submissive roles in marital relationships. Walker (1979) suggests that these victims of domestic violence typically have low self-esteem, chronic anxiety, learned helplessness, denial, shame, guilt, and psychosomatic complaints. Many women are withdrawn, depressed, and use denial to alleviate high tension levels. Johnson (1979) states that these dependent women tend to be high suicide risks.

Depression is also theorized to result from an individual's own misinterpretation of losses and life events. That depressed women tend to see themselves and the world around them in a negative manner is consistent with Beck's (1978) cognitive theory. For example, their adjustment to aging in the American youth-oriented society, where aging is not accepted (Chenitz, 1979) and where negative stereotyping of aging abounds (Emery, 1981). Women's attitudes toward themselves reveal low self-esteem and fears of failure (Bardwick, 1978; Horney, 1967), passivity and dependency (Kagan and Moss, 1971; Cooperstock, 1979), and a tendency to be self-critical (Lowenthal and Chiriboga, 1972). All these symptoms are common to the syndrome of subclinical depression (Beck *et al.*, 1979).

Treatment and Prevention

There are two concerns that remain with treatment and prevention issues. One is that traditional treatment approaches by male therapists perpetuate the passivity and negative self-image of women (Weissman and Klerman, 1977). The other is that while there are numerous programmes to treat depression, treatment usually begins after the depression has reached a serious level. This lack of early identification and intervention does not support nursing's commitment to prevention and health maintenance. Regarding the sex role stereotyping, Broverman *et al.* (1970) concluded that professional therapists have described women clients as dependent, submissive, highly emotional, and less able to make important decisions than men. Brown and Hellinger (1975) found female therapists to have more understanding attitudes toward women patients. Kjervik and Palta (1978) identified the psychiatric nurse as the professional therapist who was least likely to hold stereotypic attitudes toward women.

Rationale for a Nurse-facilitated Group Intervention

The apparent centrality of psychosocial factors to depression in women suggests that much might be done through early identification and treatment of symptoms through psychotherapeutic intervention. Once these women have been identified in urban and rural areas, growth-support groups can be established. At minimal expense these groups may provide the support necessary to develop and establish successful coping strategies for women while preventing more serious depression (Gordon and LeDray, 1984).

A group approach can be far superior to individual treatment for women in that it allows contact with peers who are likely to be dealing with some of the same role conflicts (Maykowsky, 1980). Coping strategies can be tested and shared within the supportive, safe environment of a group. These groups have been recognized as especially important in helping to lower the acknowledged sense of helplessness, powerlessness, and isolation of women living in communities (Davis, 1977). In 1981 van Servellen and Dull identified group therapy as an effective medium to promote positive change in self-esteem of depressed women. Dinnauer *et al.* (1981) emphasize the strength of groups as providing an important structure for women's social learning. Gallese and Treuting (1981) state that a women's group 'can be a lifesaver' for women feeling overwhelming stress, such as rape victims. The value of these groups goes far beyond its original purpose and provides the individuals with a sense of community (Back and Taylor, 1976).

Current literature has supported the professional nurse (minimum: baccalaureate prepared) as a facilitator of women's support groups. Loomis (1979) expected these nurses would function well as group leaders with their preparation in group dynamics and communication skills. Professional nurses (of whom 97.2 per cent in America are women) are the logical primary therapeutic change-agents in facilitating effective women's group for the following reasons.

1   They are traditionally accepted by women as trusted, caring, and helpful health professionals.
2   Academically prepared, they understand both the physiological and psychological aspects of women.
3   They appreciate the women's significant influence and role within the family system.
4   They empathize with, rather than stereotype, the women's current problems within society.
5   They serve as a positive role model for women (Gordon, 1982, note 1).

Braillier (1980) stresses the need for holistic health practice in the expanding role of the professional nurse. She feels nurses are 'ideal' resources to practice the holistic health approach since they deal with mind–body–spiritual aspects with relative ease. Professional nurses are committed to health maintenance and prevention. The efficacy for involving the client as an active participant in this emerging holistic health movement across America has been stated by Tubesing *et al.* (1977).

Results of Preliminary Studies in the United States

1979 Pilot Study

This pilot study of 19 mildly depressed women (40–60 years of age) was carried out in a midwestern city. A 10-week (90 minute per session) support group was led by two professional nurses. The volunteers were assigned to experimental and control groups and were pre- and post-tested with a battery of psychological tests. Group sessions with the nine women in the experimental group were taped. These tapes were analysed independently by three nurses (psychiatric-clinical specialists) for evidence of themes and cohesiveness (Gordon, 1982, note 1.)

Findings

1 Data on a questionnaire revealed that 36 per cent of these middle-aged women coped with daily problems using tranquillizers and that they felt justified in using alcohol when lonely.

2 Statistics were significant in that women in the experimental (treatment) group did show more improvement in the area of self-esteem, and were less depressed at the end of the group sessions than those in the control group. This group of women have continued their group experience; they still meet by themselves weekly having formed strong bonds of support and friendship.

3 Ten weeks of group sessions were found to be too few in number to resolve many problems shared by the women.

4 Tape recordings analysed after experimental group sessions revealed cohesiveness and theme examples as described below.

Session 1 Frustration of being middle-aged, 'society's throw-a-ways', anger at impatient, bored physicians for lack of understanding, help. Hostility toward men for controlling their lives.

Session 2 Feelings that 'life is scary because the rules have changed'; aware of their dependency on their husbands but feared divorce and 'going it alone'. They asked, 'where is the reward for raising children?' Anger at nurse leaders: 'you are too young to understand our problems.'

Session 3 Fears and disappointment of living with their husband's anger, his inability to cope or achieve on his job, his dependency on her. 'We've been taught to stuff our feelings, to always keep peace.' They had sad feelings of the lack of closeness to their husbands and children.

Session 4 Feelings of powerlessness, anger, loneliness, ambivalence about feeling guilty for being selfish, of putting themselves first. 'We try so hard.'

Session 5 Feelings of failure as mothers: 'the children didn't turn out as we expected and hoped.' Awareness of lack of training for jobs, fears of losing the family if they expressed their feelings of anger now after long years of marriage.

Session 6 Guilt feelings over poor relationships with their husbands; not wanting to be their husband's 'mother'; fear of loss of children's love and attention as they leave home; sexual problems with husband.

Session 7 Discouragement: men have the power, women are not valued in the job market; lack of status and respect for the housewife; fears of decreased physical attractiveness.

Section 8 Fears of cancer; need for more informatiion on menopause; afraid to try college courses as the competition is 'too tough'.

Session 9 Anger at themselves for catering to their demanding husbands: 'we are all raised to be our husband's maid'. For example, one stated: 'my husband is an executive in the second largest corporation in USA and I still butter his toast and polish his shoes!' Anxiety at the termination of groups, 'we have so much more to resolve'.

Session 10 Overwhelmed by problems of caring for aging parents. Empathy for each other; feelings of sadness and disappointment that the group is ended.

1981 Replicated Study

This replicated study of 19 mildly depressed women (40–60 years of age) was carried out in the same midwestern city. The treatment consisted of 14 weekly (2-hour) group sessions led by two professional nurses. Pre/post-testing compared nine women assigned to the structured experimental group and with ten women assigned to the no-treatment, control group (Gordon and LeDray, 1984, note 2).

Findings

1 Women who attended the group sessions showed significant reduction in depression and a significant increase in self-esteem at post-testing. In addition they showed high attendance and commitment to the group.
2 Women in the no-treatment group also showed some reduction in their depression over the 14-week period. This finding supports the notion that mild depression may lift over a period of 6 to 8 weeks.

Implications

1 Professional nurses appear to be effective facilitators of depressed women's groups.
2 Replication of the study should include moderately depressed women.

Description of 1983 Study of Depressed Women in Great Britain

Interest by the author (principle investigator) to replicate her study in England came about after the many positive relationships she had while visiting nurses in educational and hospital settings across Britain over the past decade. The similarities of the people, their language, and culture were important variables enhancing the idea of the study. The generous invitation by Jack Hayward, Head of the Department of Nursing Studies, to conduct the study at Chelsea College, University of London, was perhaps the most important incentive of all. The warm, friendly atmosphere provided by the helpful nursing faculty, staff, and students was highly conducive in making this author's experience there not only fulfilling but one of total enjoyment.

Aim of Study

The purpose of the study was to evaluate the effectiveness of a nurse-facilitated group intervention in the alleviation of depression in women of Great Britain.

Methodology

The Samples

Twenty women, 40 to 60 years of age, were selected for the study. These subjects had been recruited though a public service radio broadcast (BBC airwaves) seeking depressed women as participants. Preliminary screening took place during the eight-minute early morning public announcement by Gordon that in order for women to be eligible for the study they needed to be 40 to 60 years of age, they must speak English, and they should not presently be seeing a counsellor or psychiatrist. There was an overwhelming response to the broadcast from hundreds of women not only living in England but in areas as widespread as Wales, Belgium, Scotland, and France. The University of London's phone lines were flooded with calls, confirming the author's belief that depression in women is extensive. Over 200 women came to Chelsea College to meetings giving information about the study. Six meetings were scheduled at various hours of the week (i.e. Tuesdays 10 am, 3 pm, and 7 pm; Fridays 10 am, 3 pm and 7 pm) to fit the plans of mothers and working women. Most women were working and came to the 7 pm meetings. Gordon (principle investigator) met the women in a large classroom where introductions were made and an overview of the study was given. Many women aged 20 to 30 years came to learn about the study and were disappointed that they were unable to participate until further group experiences were available. They shared feelings of depression. All interested women ($n = 119$) who met the criteria were assigned a code number, filled out a demographic questionnaire, signed a consent form, and were given two additional tests to further help the investigator screen these volunteers. The Beck Depression Inventory (Beck, 1978) and the SCL-90-R (Derogatis, 1976) were administered. Eighty-one women who scored 14–26 on the Beck test, indicating they were mildly to moderately depressed and who were also within 'normal limits' on the SCL-90-R (therefore were not psychotic, psychopathic or suicidal) were eligible to be group members. However, the study could only include 20 women, therefore the need for random selection was indicated. All (81) code numbers were placed in a box and the first ten numbers drawn out by a visiting psychologist were assigned to the control group, the second ten code numbers pulled out by this same psychologist were assigned to the experimental group. The following week all women who came to the information meeting were informed by letter of their inclusion or exclusion in the study. Eight women who showed no depression on the Beck's test were thanked but dismissed. Thirty women who showed severe depression on the Beck's test were given information about professional resource help. Of these thirty women, six were found to be most severely depressed and the investigator informed them by telephone that their initial tests indicated that they were very depressed. The women confirmed these test results and were cooperative about seeing their general practitioner the next day. All reported back to Gordon that they had been given medication and were under the direct supervision of their physicians.

Of the twenty selected subjects, all women were white, upper middle class, with a mean age of 51 years. Eight women were married and had children, while one was divorced, five were separated, four were single, and two were widowed. Twelve women were working, one was unemployed, while seven were homemakers. Demographic differences in the experimental and control groups appeared incidental regarding age, marital status, working full-time or part-time.

Instruments Used in the Study

For selection of subjects

Beck depression inventory This inventory (Beck 1978) is a 21-item, self-report measure (range = 0–63) used to measure level of depression. The internal consistency and validity of this widely used instrument has been well documented (Beck and Beamesderfer, 1974; Shaw, 1977). The score of 14–22 is in the mild-moderate depressed range and was chosen to obtain a sample of subjects.

Test-retest stability (97 cases) over a 1 week interval was high (r's = 0.86 to 0.93) and the measure appears sensitive to spontaneous or treatment related change (Beck, 1972). There was a correlation coefficient of 0.75 between the Beck test and Hamilton Rating Scale (Schwab *et al.*, 1967). The instrument was highly effective in discriminating between depression and anxiety (Beck, 1978).

The SCL-90-R inventory This inventory (Derogatis 1976) is a 90 item self-report measure (norm T score = 50, SC = 10) used to screen for pathology and suicide risk. Designed to reflect nine psychological symptoms (obsessive-compulsive, somatization, paranoid ideation, psychoticism, depression, anxiety, hostility, phobic anxiety, and interpersonal sensitivity) seen in psychiatric patients. Measures of internal consistency were obtained from 219 hospitalized volunteers. Alpha coefficients ranged from 0.77 to 0.90 for the dimension scores. Test-retest coefficient for 94 psychiatric outpatients (over a 1 week interval) ranged from 0.80 to 0.90. The SCL-90-R correlated high 0.88 with the Minnesota Multiphasic Personality Inventory. With the Middlesex Hospital Questionnaire, six symptom dimensions were contrasted, aggregate score correlation was 0.92 (Derogatis, 1976). The SCL-90-R was chosen as the one-time assessment measure for these depressed women because of the need to eliminate from the study those who did show symptoms of psychosis, psychopathology, and suicide risk.

Pre- and post-test
(Comparison Of Control–Experimental Groups)

Coopersmith's self-esteem inventory This inventory (Ryden 1978) is a 58-item self-report used to measure self-esteem in adult subjects. Test was found to have a test-retest reliability of 0.80 for 32 women over periods of 6 to 58 weeks. The high level of stability over a period of 58 weeks reinforces the idea that the evalutive aspect of one's concept of self, as reflected in self-report, has a considerable degree of consistency over time. Because self-esteem may be related to a person's depression, Ryden's modification of the Coopersmith's self-esteem inventory was chosen to measure the subject's self-esteem.

The social adjustment self-report The SAS (Weissman and Paykel, 1974) is a 42-item instrument that measures overall social adjustment as well as performance in six major areas of functioning: work, family, social roles, etc. Self-report results based on 76 depressed out-patients were comparable to those obtained from relatives as well as by a rater who interviewed the patient directly. This measure was validated using depressed out-patients and is capable of discriminating between recovered patients and those in acute stages of illness. Validity data show that the instrument correlates highly with independent ratings of overall social adjustment made by mental health professionals ($r = 0.72$) and by significant others ($r = 0.74$). The SAS is also sensitive to change and yields significant differences in scores before and after treatment (Bothwell and Weissman, 1977).

Life experience survey The purpose of the LES (Sarason *et al.*, 1978) is to measure life changes. Advantages of this 57-item measure are that it allows for separation of positive and negative life experiences as well as individualized ratings of the impact of events. Test-retest reliability (at 5–6 weeks) is 0.56–0.88. Correlations with social desirability were −0.05 to 0.01 showing good discriminative validity. Correlations with illness, although low (0.3–0.4), are consistent with other stress measures. The LES was chosen for this study to help identify and measure stress areas of women subjects.

The young loneliness inventory The YLS (Young, 1981) is a 19 item self-report inventory used to diagnose the severity of recent loneliness. Various test items assess the client's relationship with friends and close family members during a given period of time, by rating on a scale of 0 (low) to 3 (high) the *frequency, disclosure, caring,* and *physical intimacy* they experienced in each relationship. Young establishes cutting scores as 8–9 (normal), 10–18 (mild), 19–29 moderate to severe, 30 high, and 50 as a very high degree of loneliness. The YLS has been tested for reliability and validity with both out-patient, college, and university populations. In assessing reliability, measures of consistency were obtained with these populations. Alpha coefficients ranged from 0.78 in the college to 80 in the university, to 0.84 in the mood clinic, and were considered reasonably high.

Beck depression inventory— 'significant other' form The BDI has been adapted for completion by significant other(s) of the identified patient (Hollon, 1980). All 21 items from the original inventory have been left intact other than being worded in third person, and scoring principles are identical to those for the self-report form. While little validity data are yet available for the 'significant other' form of the BDI, initial information indicated that test provides a reasonably satisfactory means of assessing depression.

Pre/Post-testing

All subjects (N-20) were given the five self-report tests described (Coopersmith's Self-Esteem, Weissman's Social Adjustment Scale, Young's Loneliness Scale, Sarason's Life Experience Survey, and the Beck Depression test filled out by a 'significant other') before the first group session started and after the fourteenth group session was over. Test scores from the control group and experimental groups were compared and changes in levels of depression, self-esteem and loneliness, etc., were analysed.

Procedure

Group Sessions

After meeting screening criteria (over radio and at the information meeting) subjects were randomly assigned to either the experimental (treatment, $n = 10$) or control (no-treatment, $n = 10$) condition. The treatment consisted of 14 weekly (2-hour) group sessions led by two professional nurses with group experience (one psychiatric nurse expert came highly recommended from Maudsley Hospital, London, one nurse with a master's degree in psychiatric nursing came from USA). These nurses were briefly orientated on the structured group intervention, which utilized a holistic health approach with concepts from the cognitive–behaviour–affective models. The nurse facilitators were provided with a training manual the contents of which included group dynamics, reinforcement theory, and evaluation of group process. Lecture content with specific objectives and discussion questions for each of the fourteen group sessions was also included in the training manual (Gordon, 1982, note 3).

The Experimental Group

Women in the experimental group chose to meet at 7–9 pm on Monday evenings in a comfortable room at Chelsea College (May–August 1983). The setting was located in a convenient, safe area of London. Some women came by car but most of them came by bus or subway trains.

During the first two sessions each woman was given equal time to 'tell her story'. After that second session repeated recounting of problems was not encouraged. The structure of group sessions devoted the first hour to lecture, education, and discussion, while the second hour was spent in activities related to the session topic. Each woman was provided with a workbook (Gordon, 1982, note 3) and was expected to come to the group sessions with assigned homework completed. Weekly topics included content found in the women's workbook: goal setting, signs and symptoms of depression, cognitions and feelings, self-worth, building relationships, communication skills, assertiveness, conflict management and decision making, stress, relaxation, exercise, nutrition, menstruation/menopause, and strength building.

All group sessions were tape-recorded for the first three sessions but this was discontinued due to inability to hear voices clearly. The women were delighted to see the tape-recorder removed.

The Control Group

Women assigned to the control condition received no intervention between pre- and post-testing. At the first information meeting they had been asked to refrain from joining other therapy groups or seeking counselling while the study was going on unless necessary. Eight women in the control condition expressed a desire to be included in later group sessions if others were to be offered.

Results

Analysis of the Data

There were no significant mean pre-treatment differences between the two treatment conditions on any of the five self-report tests, indicating that the randomization procedure was successful.

Because estimation of 'raw change' scores as measures of effectiveness of a treatment is subject to difficulties in interpretation (Cronbach and Furby, 1970), the Cohen and Cohen (1975) procedure for analysis of partial variance was used to assess the effectiveness of the treatment programme.

Statistically significant post-test differences between the control and treatment groups were demonstrated for depression, self-esteem, and hopelessness. Over 35 per cent of the variance in post-test depression scores was linearly accounted for by the pre-test depression scores. Once the effects of pre-test were removed, the treatment condition accounted for approximately 40.4 per cent of the variance in regressed change in depression from pre-test to post-test $(F=(1,17)=11.52, \ p<0.025)$. Adjustments for unreliability of the depression measure using a reliability estimate of 0.86 also resulted in significant differences between the control and treatment groups $(F=(1,17)=13.41, \ p<0.005)$. This difference represented almost one full standard deviation difference in post-test depression scores for the two groups and a classification difference from 'mild-moderate' to 'mild' on Beck's inventory.

Statistically significant improvement in scores on Coopersmith's Self-Esteem Inventory was also demonstrated for subjects in the treatment condition in comparison to those in the control group. While 54 per cent of the variance in post-test self-esteem scores could be linearly accounted for by pre-test levels of self-esteem, approximately 58.8 per cent of the variance in regressed change from pre-test to post-test was accounted for by treatment condition $(F=(1,17)=24.23, \ p<0.001)$. Adjustments for unreliability of the self-esteem measure using 0.80 as an estimate of reliability yielded even higher statistically significant results ($F = (1,17)$ $= 56.92$, $p < 0.001$). Mean post-test scores adjusted for unreliability and pre-test performance were 63.78 for the treatment group and 48.12 for the control group. Again, the treatment group was almost one full standard deviation above the control group in post-test self-esteem level.

Feelings of hopelessness were also significantly reduced between pre-test and post-test for the treatment subjects, whereas there was an increase in these feelings for the control group over the same period. Over 20 per cent of the variance in post-test hopelessness scores was accounted for by pre-test feelings of hopelessness and 45.2 per cent of the variance in regressed change in hopelessness scores was accounted for by the treatment manipulation ($F = (1,17) = 14.01$, $p < 0.005$). No direct reliability estimates for the Beck Hopelessness Scale were available so a reliability of 0.80 was assumed. Adjustments to the analysis based upon this level of reliability resulted in higher levels of statistical significance ($F = (1,17) = 20.81$, $p < 0.001$). Subjects in the treatment group ($X = 5.76$) scored over six units below the subjects in the control group ($X = 11.82$). This difference between treatment and control groups represented over one standard deviation difference in performance.

Similar analyses were applied to the remaining dependent measures. No statistically significant differences between control and treatment groups on the post-test measures for loneliness, depression as rated by a significant other, social adjustment or anxiety level were observed. Perhaps the 14-week time interval for the study was not a sufficient time period to observe significant changes on these variables. Also, the significant other form of the Beck Depression Inventory is not as valid as the self-report form and, generally, measures of depression by significant others tend to underestimate self-report measures of depression. Both of these could have affected the results of the study.

The findings suggest that nurse-facilitated groups do provide a therapeutic value to moderately depressed women. The 14-week time interval was sufficient to demonstrate improvement in subjects' feelings of self-esteem and reduction in their feelings of depression and hopelessness. It seems reasonable that improvement in a woman's feelings of self-esteem and self-concept could potentially stress other aspects of her life as she learned to cope with her new sense of being and with others in her life. Also, it is possible that others, especially significant others in her life, must also learn to adapt to a woman with higher feelings of self-esteem. Perhaps this accounts for the lack of significant change in the feelings of loneliness, social adjustment, and anxiety observed in this study. Further studies should investigate this possibility.

Observations of Women in Group by Nurse-facilitators

Observation notes were carefully written by both nurse group-facilitators after each session. The date, the number of members present, and the reactions of members relating to lateness or absence of peers were recorded in notebooks. Individual verbal/non-verbal behaviour was described, as well as indications of group stages, themes, and cohesiveness observed. The group met during Summer 1983. The notebooks were mailed to the author (principle investigator) in America for analysis after group sessions were over.

The wealth of information emerging from the content of the notebooks was too great to be included in this single chapter, however specific data observed during each session is described. Names have been changed for confidentiality. In comparing the responses of the American women and the British women, it seems that the American women appeared to be less reserved, more open to share unacceptable feelings earlier in sessions. British women seemed to need more support to be aware of their deeper feelings and to reveal life experiences. They also were extremely sensitive to each other's feelings, offering advice and help. There was no evidence in the British women's group of a power struggle with the nurse leaders as was apparent in the American women's group.

Condensed Data in Notebooks

The information presented from the 14 sessions is given in note form.

Session 1

All women arrived on time, except Diane who had 'forgotten' about a previous engagement. All members were well dressed, neat. They looked like serious business women as introductions were made. Everyone was polite and interested. During the nurse's explanation of expectations for group leaders and members, rules of confidentiality etc., most women sat with folded arms and guarded facial expressions. After tea and coffee, the members seemed to feel more relaxed with the two nurses gently inviting more trust. Many questions indicating anxiety about their own expectations of the group sessions arose. There was denial of feelings, i.e. 'Well, there really isn't much to talk about,' or 'Oh, I couldn't talk about anger because I have never felt it.' Two women felt there was danger in becoming 'too introspective'. Several shared their loathing of lies. Themes: mistrust, anger, sadness, and some wonder of 'how "things" at home can really change'.

Session 2

All women were punctual. With little hesitation they went into talking about their life problems. There were 'moving' moments as the women revealed their suffering and how they had suppressed a lot of their own feelings for the 'good of the family'. Support for each other was evident, i.e. 'Yes, I know what you mean, I felt that pain too when my children left home.' Women appeared more positive, they said they looked forward to coming to the group, i.e. 'Its good that there are others we can talk to.' Themes: marriage vs career, the freedom and the frustrations of living alone. Stages: trust, some cohesiveness, i.e. use of 'we' instead of 'me'.

Session 3

Nearly everyone was talking at once. Much discussion, 'advice giving'. The group felt very charged and intense, with great sharing of deep losses, personal failures in life. Several spoke of painful separation from family when sent to boarding schools. Facilitators felt exhausted after the session and were concerned that 'too much was shared too early'.

Session 4

The group was dominated by Lisa who spent a great deal of time on frivolous events in her life; there was much chit-chat and unheeded advice giving. Nurses facilitators found themselves irritated that the group was not 'moving', that there seemed to be a conscious avoidance of sharing deep feelings . . . perhaps too painful from the last session. Nurses did intervene, taking control of the storytelling and the women grew thoughtful. Themes: loneliness, feelings of low self-worth, loss of male companionship.

Session 5

Three members were absent. The group appeared quiet, serious, more of a 'working' group. More intimacy emerged, e.g. how they felt powerless in marital relationships with their husbands who 'did what they wanted'. Tremendous denial of their anger toward others. They tended to blame themselves that their children did not meet their expectations, that they were concerned and hurt how their children reacted to relatives, friends. Stage: intimacy.

Session 6

Again much 'advice giving' (how to lose weight etc.) was apparent, and facilitators needed to get the group back to talking about the assigned homework on discussing feelings. It was a very productive session with much clarification of negative and positive feelings, of how 'should', 'ought', 'must' thinking causes their feelings of hopelessness. One woman shared how hard it was being the 'other' woman in a relationship and received support and understanding.

Session 7

Homework assignment related to learning how difficult it was to learn how to be assertive. They said they were 'brought up' to be nice, lovely ladies and it was easier to remain passive. They found it most difficult to be aggressive and nearly impossible to be assertive. Some 'pairing off' by group members, some non-direct hostility toward a domineering member.

Session 8

'Entire group came looking very pretty tonight', wrote one nurse facilitator. The women initiated discussion on the value of the group. One woman had been turned down twice that week for jobs, but had looked forward to coming to the group for support. Much sincere feedback and support was evident. Karen said she could take what she learned in each group session and apply it daily. Facilitators felt sad and shared these feelings with the group: many women had said that this group was the 'only' place they felt they could speak freely and easily. Stage: cohesiveness, group running itself.

Session 9

Vera was leaving the group for a new job in Southeast Asia. Fears and anxieties were expressed by Vera. All members told her they were happy for her, sad for themselves, and a bit envious of her new adventure. She thanked them for their caring and was taking her Women's Workbook with her. Again when advice was given to various members Elaine expressed frustration that members weren't allowing self-decision-making. Reactions were highly defended and difficult. Facilitators felt the group seemed blocked and permitted power struggles.

Session 10

No absences. Group members seemed much more serious, using workbooks, reflecting more on their own reactions to daily stress. Both nurses wrote: 'These women are bright, of high intelligence, and gain insight with relative ease.' Lisa appears to have learned constructive ways of dealing with conflicts regarding her employer. More women said they had more energy and more interest in life.

Session 11

Much discussion on feelings of failures as mothers. Expressions of anger, guilt. There was beginning talk about how sad it was that the group would soon come to an end. Reflections about Vera separating from them to go to Asia brought out an atmosphere of sombre mellowness. Peggy shared for the first time that she was chemically dependent. The group was surprised at this, but supported her for continuing to come to group and work on her low self-esteem. Women went on to discuss the problem of being divorced and having no job skills. (This is a similiar problem of middle-aged women in the United States.)

Session 12

Much talk of guilt when they say 'no' to doing favours for others and what to do about that guilt. Some pressure on facilitators to come up with answers. Many spoke of resistance to physical exercise. Some insight on how they resist change throughout their lives and it brings them depression. 'It is hard to change our habits.' Good discussion on the fears of taking risks to change. Definite cohesiveness between members . . . women see the facilitators as members.

Session 13

Discussion of menstruation and menopause evoked feelings of the loss of childbearing ability for some members. Support was given to each other. Others spoke of the pains of motherhood. One shared how much the group had helped her to see her children more objectively, to give them freedom to be adults, and be more accepting of her son and his 'unconventional' behaviour. She said she felt much happier in herself and that she couldn't have achieved that without help of the group. Afterwards group facilitators felt frustrated because there had not been enough time to discuss the sexual conflicts alluded to by several members.

Session 14

The last group centred on sexuality: both strategies for building positive and intimate sexual relationships, as well as sources for sexual conflict were discussed. Some women described sexual conflicts with their lovers or husbands, others explained their relationships lacked all sexual intimacy. It was interesting to observe how relaxed most of the women were discussing such personal problems. The last half hour of this session was used for group evaluation and feedback. The women felt sad that it was their last group because they felt that they had learned to trust and confide in each other. One member said she had never considered that the group would end. There was a consensus of opinion by all members and facilitators that the number of group meetings should be expanded to at least 20 sessions, so that the women would have more time to learn and test the coping skills they needed in meeting their daily problems. Facilitators felt more time was needed for termination. All the women described the groups as helpful, insightful, and supportive. They hoped to remain in touch with each other and there was an exchange of addresses. The women also gave cards and gifts to the nurses, who felt it was a wonderful experience for them. All left with much handshaking, some hugging, and tear-filled eyes.

Summary and Implications for Nursing

The widespread incidence of depression in women is identified as a major health problem in the world today. Prominent researchers report that women are twice as likely as men to suffer from depression. This chapter provides documentation of the stress factors that occur in women's daily lives which stem from social, family, and cultural demands on them. Women are still regarded as 'second-class' citizens with society's expectation that they are caretakers of men and children first while their own potential for self-actualization is disregarded. A consequence of this lack of recognition decreases women's self-fulfilment and self-worth. Women are the most underutilized talent in the world. Their sensitivity, creativeness, management skills, and enduring strength in crisis is taken for granted and undervalued. As a result they have feelings of frustration, inadequacy, and low self-esteem. Close relationships with significant others are of utmost importance to women. It is around attachment issues, more than any other sorts of issues, that depressive episodes in women tend to emerge. Women invest highly in intimate relationships with men and their children and to fail in those relationships, or to have them end becomes equated with failing in everything. Conflicts with husbands, children, in-laws, and lovers are cited by women as principal causes for their depression. Depressed women in America have increased medical costs due to their repeated visits to physicians for psychosomatic complaints, chemical dependency, unnecessary gynaecological surgery, and high admissions to psychiatric hospital units. Due to the rising cost of health care, treatment approaches need to be efficacious, safe and cost-effective.

A description of three research studies utilizing a nursing intervention model of treatment designed by the author has been presented. Two preliminary studies were conducted in the United States with thirty-eight women (40–60 years of age) as subjects. The purpose of the studies was to evaluate the effectiveness of a group intervention facilitated by professional nurses in alleviating depression in women. Pre/post-testing revealed that women who attended the structured group sessions showed a significant reduction in depression and a significant increase in self-esteem. In addition the participants' support and commitment to the group was demonstrated by high attendance to group sessions and their continued networking after the group session were over. Findings support the view that mild depression may lift over a period of 6–8 weeks and that replication of the study should include moderately depressed women.

The third study, a replication of the intervention model, was conducted in the University of London with twenty moderately depressed middle-aged women. These volunteers were randomly selected and assigned to either the experimental or control condition. The treatment consisted of 14 weekly (2-hour) structured group sessions led by two professional nurses in London. Detailed description of methodology, findings as well as nurses' observation by the group's nurse-facilitators are included in the chapter. Again, statistically significant post-test differences between control and experimental groups were demonstrated for depression, self-esteem and hopelessness.

The following conclusions emerge:

1   Professional nurses (baccalaureate graduates) tend to be effective facilitators of depressed women's groups. Nurses' abilities to help women has been substantiated in these studies in the USA and the UK.
2   That coping strategies for women can be taught, tested and shared within a supportive group atmosphere.
3   That replication of the intervention model with increased numbers of women of a variety of ages and background could be useful future nursing research.

The significance of the intervention model is:

1   to help women cope effectively, take an active role in their own health;
2   to prevent possible severe depression in women;
3   to gain data about the complex phenomena of depression in women;
4   to strengthen the family unit by increased self-esteem of women.

Use of this approach by nurses already available in the community to provide women this assistance (by use of provided instruction manuals for the group facilitators as well as for each woman) could also reduce health care costs.

Presently a replication of the study will be conducted over three years in USA involving 300 moderately depressed women as participants. *The Women's Workbook* and the *Group Facilitator Manual* are being revised by the author to cover twenty group sessions and suggested additional content (i.e. areas on human sexuality, loss, and grief).

Acknowledgments

The author wishes to acknowledge the excellent professional nurses who facilitated the women's group sessions at Chelsea College, University of London: Beatrice Stevens, SRN, RMN, Psychiatric Nurse Clinical Specialist, Maudsley Hospital, London, and Marion Talmadge Reed, BSN, MN, Psychiatric Nurse Clinical Specialist from Boston College and Emory University, Atlanta, Georgia, USA, presently working in Community Mental Health, London.

The Minnesota research projects were supported in part by the Graduate School, University of Minnesota (Grant No. 452-0325-4909-02, July 1980-1981) and the Archie D. and Bertha Walker Foundation, Minneapolis, Minnesota (1979). The Study at Chelsea College, University of London, was partially funded by The Burroughs Wellcome Fund, Research Triangle Park, North Carolina, USA and National Institute of Health, Fogarty International Scholarship, Bethesda, Maryland, USA.

Reference Notes

1.   Gordon, V. C. (1982). Themes and cohesiveness observed in depressed women's support group. *Issues in Mental Health Nursing*, **4**, 115–125.
2.   Gordon, V. C. and Ledray, L. (1984). 'The alleviation of subclinical depression in women of middle years', (In Press).
3.   Gordon, V. C. (1982). The *Nurse Facilitator Manual* and participant's *Women's Workbook* developed for this project will be available from the author.

References

Back, K. W. and Taylor, R. (1976). Self-help groups: tool or symbol? *Journal of Applied Behavioural Science*, 12, 295–309.

Bardwick, J. M. (1978). Middle age and a sense of future. *Merrill-Palmer Quarterly*, 24, 130–136.

Barrett, N. (1979). Women in the job market: occupations, earnings and career opportunities, in R. Smith (Ed.), *The Subtle Revolution: Women at Work*. Urban Institute, Washington, D. C.

Bart, P. B. (1971). Depression in middle-aged Women, in V. Gomich and B. Moran (Eds), *Women in Sexist Society*. Basic Books, New York, 163–186.

Beck, A. T. (1972). Measuring depression: the depression inventory. In T. A. Williams, M. N. Katz and J. A. Shield (Eds), *Recent Advances in the Psychobiology of the Depressive Illnesses*. Government Printing Office, Washington, D.C.

Beck, A. T. (1978). *Depression: Causes and Treatment*. University of Pennsylvania Press, Philadelphia, P.A., 12–43, 186–207.

Beck, A. T. and Beamesderfer, A. (1974). Assessment of depression, the depression inventories, in P. Pichot (Ed.), *Psychological Measurements in Psychopharmacology and Modern Pharmacopsychiatry*, vol. 7. Karger, Basle, Switzerland.

Beck, A. T., Rush, A. J., Shaw, B. F., and Emery G. (1979). *Cognitive Therapy of Depression*, Guilford Press, New York.

Belle, D. (1982). *Lives in Stress: Women and Depression*. Sage Publications, Beverly Hills, CA.

Bothwell, S. and Weissman, M. (1977). Social impairments four years after an acute depressive episode. *American Journal of Orthopsychiatry*, 47, 231–237.

Brailler, L. (1980). Holistic health practice: expanding the role of the psychiatric-mental health nurse, in J. Lancaster (Ed.), *Community Mental Health Nursing*. Mosby, New York.

Broverman, I. K., Broverman, D., Clarkson, F. E., Rosendrantz, P., and Vogel, S. R. (1970). Sex-role stereotypes and clinical judgments of mental health. *Journal of Counseling and Clinical Psychology*, 34, 1–7.

Brown, C. R. and Hellinger, M. L. (1975). Therapists' attitudes toward women. *Social Work*, 21, 266–270.

Brown, G. W., Bhrolchain M. N., and Harris, T. (1975). Social class and psychiatric disturbance among women in an urban population. *Sociology*, 9, 225–254.

Carmen, E., Russo, N. F., and Miller, J. B. (1981). Inequality and women's mental health: an overview. *American Journal of Psychiatry*, 138, 1319–1330.

Chenitz, W. C. (1979). Primary depression in older women: are current theories and treatment of depression relevant to this age group? *Journal of Psychiatric Nursing and Mental Health Services*, 17–23.

Cherlin, A. J. (1981). *Marriage, Divorce, Remarriage*. Harvard University Press, Boston, MA.

Chodoff, P. (1972). The depressive personality. *Archives of General Psychiatry*, 27, 666–673.

Claerhout, S., Elder, J., and Carolyn, J. (1982). Problem-solving skills of rural battered women. *American Journal of Community Psychology*, 10 (5), 605–606.

Clayton, P. J., Martin, S., Davis, M., and Wochnik, E. (1980). Mood disorders in women professionals. *Journal of Affective Disorders*, **2**, 37–46.

Cohen, J. and Cohen, P. (1975). *Applied Multiple Regression/Correlation Analysis for the Behavioral Sciences*, Wiley, New York, 378–393.

Cooperstock, R. (1979). A review of women's psychotropic drug use. *Canadian Journal of Psychiatry*, **24**, 29–34.

Cronbach, L. J. and Furby, L. (1970). How should we measure 'change' — or should we?, *Psychological Bulletin*, **74**, 68–80.

Curlee, Joan. (1969). *Alcoholism and the 'empty nest'*. Bulletin of Menninger Clinic, **33**, 165–170.

Davis, S. M. (1977). Women's liberation groups as a primary preventive mental health strategy. *Community Mental Health Journal*, **13**, 219–228.

Dohrenwend, B. S. (1973). Social status and stressful life events. *Journal of Personality and Social Psychology*, **28**, 225–235.

Derogatis, L. (1976). *SCL-90 (Revised Version) Manual-1*. Johns Hopkins University School of Medicine, Baltimore, Md. 21205.

Dinnauer, L., Miller, M., and Frankforter, M. (1981). Implementation strategies for an inpatient woman's support group. *Journal of Psychiatric Nursing and Mental Health Services*, **19**, 13–16.

Editorial (1979). Hysterectomy and the quality of a woman's life. *Archives of International Medicine*, **139**, 146.

Emery, G. (1981). *A New Beginning: How You Can Change Your Life Through Cognitive Therapy*. Simon and Schuster, New York.

Fiske, D. W., Hunt, H. F., Luborsky, L., Orne, T. M., Parloff, M. B., Reiser, M. F., and Tuma, A. H. (1970). Planning of research on effectiveness of psychotherapy. *Archives of General Psychiatry*, **22**, 22.

Gallese, L. and Treuting, E. (1981). Help for rape victims through group therapy. *Journal of Psychiatric Nursing and Mental Health Services*, **19**, 20–21.

Goldberg, A. (1973). Psychotherapy of narcissistic injuries. *Archives of General Psychiatry*, **28**, 722–726.

Gordon, V. C. (1982). Themes and cohesives observed in a depressed women's support group. *Issues in Mental Health Nursing*, **4**, 115–125.

Gordon, V. and Ledray, L. (1985). Depression in women: the challenge of treatment and prevention. *Journal of Psychosocial Nursing and Mental Health Services*, **23**, 26–34.

Gordon, V. C. (1979). Women and divorce: implications for nursing care, in *Women in Stress: A Nursing Perspective*, O. O. Kjervik-Martinson (Ed.) Appleton-Century-Croft, New York, 259–276.

Gove, W. (1972). The relationship between sex roles, mental illness and marital status. *Social Forces*, **51**, 34–44.

Guttentag, Salasin, S., and Belle, D. (1980). *The Mental Health of Women*. Academic Press, New York, 21–30, 57–89.

Hirschfield, R. M. (1980). In M. Scarf (Ed.), *Unfinished Business: Pressure Points in the Lives of Women*. Ballatine Books, New York, 277.

Hollon, S. O. (1980). Beck's 'Significant Other' Form (unpublished).

Horney, Karen. (1967). *Feminine Psychology*. W. W. Norton, New York, 124–132.

Johnson, K. K. (1979). Durkheim revisited: why do women kill themselves? *Suicide and Life Threatening Behaviour*, **9**, 145–153.

Kagan, J. and Moss, H. A. (1971). Birth to maturity, in J. M. Bardwick (Ed.), *Psychology of Women*. Harper and Row, New York.

Kaslow S. (1982). Marriage and intimacy: The surprising staying power of loveless marriages. *Ladies Home Journal*, 3, 41–48.

Kivett, V. R. (1979). Religious motivation in middle age: correlates and implications. *Journal of Gerontology*, 34, 106–115.

Kjervik, D. K. and Palta, M. (1978). Sex-role stereotyping in assessments of mental health. *Nursing Research*, 27, 166–171.

LeDray, L. and Chaignot, M. (1980). Services to sexual assault victims in Hennepin County. *Evaluation and Change*, special issue, 131–134.

Lewinsohn, P., Sullivan, J., and Grosscup, S. (1982). Behavioral therapy: clinical applications, in A. J. Rush (Ed.), *Short Term Psychotherapies of Depression*. The Guilford Press, New York, 50–87.

Loomis, M. E. (1979). *Group Process for Nurses*. vol. 23, Mosby, St. Louis, Md., 146–147.

Lopata, H. Z. (1971). Widows as a minority group. *The Gerontologist*, Spring, 67–75.

Lowenthal, M. F. and Chiriboga, D. (1972). Transition to the empty nest: crisis, challenge or relief? *Archives of General Psychiatry*, 26, 8–14.

Martin, R. L., Roberts, W. V., and Clayton, P. J. (1980). Psychiatric status after hysterectomy. *Journal of the American Medical Association*, 244, 350–353.

Maykowsky, V. P. (1980). Stress and mental health of women: a discussion of research and issues, in M. Guttentag (Ed.), *The Mental Health of Women*. Academic Press, New York.

McLachlan, J. F., R. L. Walderman, D. F. Birchmore, and Marsden, L. R. (1976). Self-evaluation, role satisfaction in the woman alcoholic. *The International Journal of Addictions*, 14 (6), 809–832.

Miller, J. (1976). *Toward A New Psychology of Women*, Beacon Press, Boston, MA., 64–73.

Neuberry, P., Weissman, M., and Myers, J. (1979). Working wives and housewives: do they differ in mental status and social adjustment? *American Journal Orthopsychiatry*, 49, 282–290.

Neugarten, B., Wood, L., Krainer, R., and Loomis, B. (1963). Women's attitudes toward the menopause. *Vita Humana*, 6, 140–151.

Notman, M. (1979). Midlife concerns in women: implications of the menopause. *American Journal of Psychiatry*, 136, 1270–1274.

Notman, M., Nadelson, C., and Bennett, M. (1978). Achievement conflict in women. *Psychotherapy and Psychosomatics*, 29, 203–213.

Parloff, Morris B. (1980). Psychotherapy and research: an anaclitic depression. *Psychiatry*, 43, 280.

Pilisuk, M. and Froland, C., (1978). Kinship, social network, social support and health. *Social Science and Medicine*, 12 (B), 273–280.

Powell, B. (1977). The empty nest, employment, and psychiatric symptoms in college-educated women. *Psychology of Women Quarterly*, 2, 35–43.

Radloff, L. (1975). Sex differences in depression: the effects of occupation and marital status. *Sex Roles*, 1, 249–264.

Radloff, L., and Monroe, M. (1978). Sex differences in helplessness–with implications for depression. In Hansen L. and Rapoza, R. (Eds), *Career Development and Counseling of Women*. Thomas, Springfield, Illinois, 199–204.

Radloff, L. S. and Rae, D. (1979). Susceptibility and precipitating factors in depression: sex differences and similarities. *Journal of Abnormal Psychology*, **88**, 174–181.

Raphael, B. (1976). Psychiatric aspects of hysterectomy. In J. G. Howell (Ed.). *Modern Perspectives in the Psychiatric Aspects of Surgery*. Brunner-Mazel, New York, 425.

Ryden, M. (1978). Coopersmith self-esteem inventory (adult version). *Psychological Reports*, **43**, 1189–1980.

Sarason, I., Johnson, J., and Siegel, J. (1978). Assessing the impact of life changes: development of the Life Experiences Survey, *Journal of Consulting and Clinical Psychology*, **46**, 932–946.

Scarf, M. (1980). *Unfinished Business: Pressure Points in the Lives of Women*. Ballantine Books, New York, 442–448.

Schaef, A. W. (1981). *Women's Reality*. Winston Press, Minneapolis, MN.

Schwab, J. J., Bralow, M., and Holzer, C. (1967). A comparison of two rating scales for depression. *Journal of Clinical Psychology*, **23**, 94–96.

Seligman, M. E. (1975). *Helplessness*. W. H. Freeman, San Francisco.

Shaw, B. F. (1977). Comparison of cognitive therapy and behavior therapy in the treatment of depression. *Journal of Consulting and Clinical Psychology*, **45**, 543–551.

Shields, L. (1980). *Displaced Homemakers*. McGraw-Hill, New York.

Stevenson, J. (1977). *Issues and Crises During Middlescence*. Appleton-Century-Crofts, New York, 165, 168–186, 216.

Thurnher, M. (1976). Midlife marriage: sex differences in evaluation and perspectives. *International Journal of Aging and Human Development*, **7**, 129–135.

Tubesing, D., Holinger, P., Westberg, G., and Lichter, E. (1977). The Wholistic Health Center Project. *Medical Care*, **15**, 217–227.

Tucker, S. J. (1977). The menopause: How much soma and how much psyche? *JOGN Nursing*, **6**, 40–47.

van Keep, P. and Prill, H. (1975). Psycho-sociology of menopause and post-menopause. *Frontiers in Hormone Research*, **3**, 32–39.

van Servellen, G. and Dull, L. (1981). Group psychotherapy for depressed women: a model. *Journal of Psychiatric Nursing and Mental Health Services*, **19**, 25–30.

Walker, L. E. (1979). *The Battered Woman*. Harper and Row, New York.

Weissman, M. M. and Paykel, E. S., (1974). *The Depressed Woman*. University of Chicago Press, Chicago, Illinois.

Weissman, M. M. and Klerman, G. L. (1977). Sex differences and the epidemiology of depression. *Archives of General Psychiatry*, **34**, 98–111.

Weissman, M., Pincus, C., Radding, N., Lawrence, R., and Siegel, R. (1973). The educated housewife: mild depression and the search for work. *American Journal Orthopsychiatry*, **43** (4), 565–573.

Wittenborn, J. R. and Buhler, R. (1979). Somatic discomforts among depressed women. *Archives of General Psychiatry*, **36**, 465–471.

Wood, H. P. and Duffy, E. L. (1966). Psychological factors in alcoholic women. *American Journal of Psychiatry*, **123** (3), 341–345.

Young, J. E. (1981). Cognitive therapy and loneliness, in G. Emery, S. Hollon, and R. Bedrosian (Eds), *New Directions in Cognitive Therapy*. Guilford Press, New York, 139–159.

CHAPTER 7

Extended Study to Evaluate Nurses' Attitudes to Geriatric Psychiatry

R. GLYN JONES

Editor's Comments

This study developed because of a need in the researcher's area to plan for the redeployment of nurses from general psychiatry to psychogeriatric care as new wards and day-care facilities were developed for the increasing elderly population.

In this chapter, Glyn Jones describes some of the results from his survey of psychiatric nurses' opinions about working with the elderly mentally infirm. The majority of the large sample of nurses reported very positive attitudes towards psychogeriatric nursing, which is an interesting and perhaps surprising finding.

Introduction

After a series of discussions involving the researcher, a consultant psychiatrist, a principal clinical psychologist, and nurse managers, the following hypothesis was formulated: 'A negative view towards geriatric-psychiatry nursing areas will be found among nursing staff'.

Background

Early in 1982 a pilot study was carried out in two psychiatric hospitals in Scotland to examine nurses' attitudes towards psychogeriatric nursing. Jones and Galliard (1982) hypothesized that a uniformly negative view would be held by the nursing staff in a psychiatric hospital, but they found the opposite. The recommendation of their pilot study led to this larger scale replication in five psychiatric hospitals in Scotland.

Review of the Literature

There have been few studies of psychogeriatric nursing. In 1975 Towell published a social anthropological case study concerning the role of nurses in a psychiatric hospital including a psychogeriatric ward. The dominant concern on the psychogeriatric ward was the 'routine servicing' of patients, and while patient-centred care was held as an ideal, it was seen as impossible, due to lack of resources. There was little verbal interaction between staff and patients; and patients were regarded as depersonalized objects.

Miller (1978) attempted to evaluate the care given to demented patients in six long-stay wards. Physical care was generally adequate, but there was a lack of clear goals, communication, and overall policy. There seemed to be no attempt to individualize care. The severely demented patients spent only 34 per cent of their time in 'engaged' activities. Miller recommended the introduction of more individualized care, written objectives, and support from senior staff.

The Hospital Innovation Project (Towell and Harries, 1979) was a five-year action research study involving many projects initiated by ward staff in various areas of a psychiatric hospital. As part of the project Savage *et al.* (1979) found that nurses in a psychogeriatric ward spent more than 50 per cent of their time on physical care. Increasing staff numbers led to more physical care, but no increase in psychological care. They discussed how the Warehousing Model (Miller and Gwynne, 1974) used in the ward reinforced dependency and reduced patient autonomy.

Another study relevant to psychogeriatric care was carried out on general geriatric wards by Wells (1980). She found that learner nurses and nursing auxiliaries gave the majority of direct care, while qualified staff were occupied in administrative duties. Wells suggested that nursing was focused not on the patients but on the routine. Periods of intense rushed nursing activity alternated with periods of relative inactivity away from the patients. Wells argued that the excuse of staff shortages was a rationalization to alleviate feelings of failure. The real problem was poor organization, and a more individualized approach was needed.

A search of the literature on nurses' attitudes towards the psychogeriatric nursing service showed that little work has been done. However, there has been a great deal of research into nurses' attitudes towards various general nursing specialties. Shanley (1981) pointed out that most attitude research in the psychiatric field has been undertaken in America. In a study concerning nurses' attitudes towards mental illness, Reznikoff (1963) found that trained nurses had a more approving and less custodial attitude than nursing aides. Similarly, Appleby *et al.* (1961) found that professional members of the multidisciplinary team had less authoritarian attitudes to the mentally ill than non-professional members of the team.

Method

Design

The design of the attitude survey took the form of a one-shot exploratory study, the results of which are based upon completed questionnaires returned by the subjects. The document used consisted of a pre-coded self-completion questionnaire containing a series of statements concerning the geriatric-psychiatry nursing area.

Hospitals

Data were collected from five psychiatric hospitals in Scotland. Each hospital was built during the last century and each had several hundred beds.

Subjects

The subjects consisted of all nursing staff at the two hospitals. There were 1117 nurses employed in the hospitals of whom 910 responded, that is, a response rate of 81.5 per cent. Of the number that responded 29.2 per cent (267) were male nurses and 70.8% (643) were female nurses. The age range was from 18 to approximately 46 years. All grades of nurses and nursing auxiliaries took part in the study up to nursing officers. Senior

Table 1   Status and number of staff in the study

Grade	number
Nursing officers	25
Charge nurses	125
Staff nurses	127
Enrolled nurses	207
Student nurses	65
Pupil nurses	41
Auxiliaries	320
Total	910

nursing officers and above were excluded because of the small number of people in those positions and thus the impossibility of assuring their anonymity. The questionnaires were sent to all subjects at the same time. The number of subjects in each grade is shown in Table 1.

The Questionnaire

Data were collected using a self-completion questionnaire developed from the pilot study carried out at two of the hospitals (Jones and Galliard, 1982). The questionnaire was a five-page document. The first page consisted of an introduction to the study and instructions on completion and return of the questionnaires. It also contained an assurance of anonymity of the subject. The second page contained questions concerning personal details, such as sex, age, marital status, and time in nursing. The next page asked the subjects which psychiatric nursing areas they had worked in and their opinions of these areas. The last two pages listed 17 attitude statements pertinant to the geriatric-psychiatry nursing area. The subjects were asked to respond to each statement by placing a tick to indicate strongly agree, agree, undecided, disagree or strongly disagree. The items were precoded for computer analysis using the Statistical Package for the Social Sciences.

Discussion of Results

It was hypothesized that nurses taking part in this survey would have negative attitudes towards the geriatric-psychiatry nursing area. However, the results do not appear to support this hypothesis, but reflect those found in the pilot study. The overall response rate was 81.5 per cent and was consistently high across the five hospitals, varying from 73.7 per cent to 85.1 per cent. This suggests that nursing staff have an active interest in research concerning the geriatric-psychiatry nursing areas.

The first attitude statement was 'I find it really distressing working as a nurse on a geriatric-psychiatry ward'. A total of 88.4 per cent of the nurses disagreed or strongly disagreed with the statement leaving 11.6 per cent of the subjects who may find a certain amount of distress working on these wards. Further research into this small subgroup is needed to establish reasons for the distress of these nurses and how to alleviate it.

The second attitude statement was 'Working on a geriatric-psychiatry ward is not very challenging'. A total of 78.7 per cent of the cohort disagreed or strongly disagreed with the statement leaving 21.3 per cent of nursing staff who find this nursing area a working environment which does not present a challenge to them.

The third attitude statement was 'I prefer working in a geriatric-psychiatry setting as opposed to a general psychiatry one'. Responses to this showed a general split in the group with a substantial number undecided. Less than half, 41.2 per cent, of the group agreed or strongly agreed with the statement, illustrating that they showed a preference for geriatric-psychiatry. However, 30 per cent indicated that they would prefer to work in other areas and 28.8 per cent were undecided. The numbers reported appear to show that more psychiatric nurses would prefer to work in a geriatric-psychiatry setting than in a general psychiatry nursing area.

The fourth attitude statement was 'Working on a geriatric-psychiatry ward is interesting and personally rewarding'. A total of 78.4 per cent of the sample agreed or strongly agreed, 12.9 per cent disagreed or strongly disagreed, while 8.7 per cent remained undecided. The responses show a very positive attitude to this nursing area. It is possible that the minority of subjects who were undecided may consist of learner nurses and auxiliaries who had not worked in this nursing specialty.

The last statement was 'I am very satisfied working on a geriatric-psychiatry ward because I am making greater use of my nursing skills'. A total of 51.8 per cent of the subject group agreed or strongly agreed with the statement, 24.3 per cent disagreed, and 23.9 per cent were undecided.

The overall responses of the subjects appear not to support the initial hypothesis presented at the beginning of the study. A large proportion of the subject group seem to be completely satisfied with their position in a geriatric-psychiatry setting. However, a minority do report feeling distress in this nursing area and further studies may highlight the problems they experience and show how to remedy them. The challenges of this nursing area do not appear to deter a large percentage of the cohort in their attitudes to the area (statement 2) and they appear to show a slight preference for a geriatric-psychiatric setting as opposed to a general psychiatry setting (statement 3). The subjects appear to have sustained interest in this nursing area and gain personal reward from it (statement 4). Most subjects agree that the geriatric-psychiatry nursing area allows them greater use of their nursing skills.

These results, obtained from 910 nurses from five psychiatric hospitals in Scotland, appear to be consistent in their rejection of the hypothesis. In the pilot study it was argued that the results might have been unique to the two hospitals concerned. Since this replication and extension of the study, this caution appears to be unnecessary, as the results obtained in both this and the pilot study are consistent.

Further analysis of the results would be beneficial in showing the opinions of the different groups of nursing staff. It might thus be possible to identify the characteristics of nurses who suffer distress in the geriatric-psychiatry nursing area (statement 1) and enable further research to outline the reasons for distress and possible solutions. Further exploration of the characteristics of nurses who do not find challenge in the geriatric-psychiatry setting is needed. This might identify methods of involving those nurses in the challenges of this speciality.

The questions that arise from the minority who have negative attitudes towards geriatric-psychiatry are manifold, but a basic question is 'why?'. In future studies semi-structured interviews may be appropriate as they allow discussion and comment and may be far more revealing. Although interviews are more time consuming than postal questionnaires, the results may outweigh the time and expenditure. Through this method, the possibility of the introduction of ward-based in-service training/education programmes may enlighten nurses to the challenges and rewards of psychogeriatric care.

Conclusions

This study of 910 nurses in five Scottish psychaitric hospitals has revealed positive attitudes towards the geriatric-psychiatry nursing area. These results appear to refute the popular belief that nurses dislike working with the elderly mentally infirm. The study has supported the results of an earlier pilot study (Jones and Galliard, 1982).

Note Copies of the questionnaires are available from the author at Murray Royal Hospital, Muirhall Road, Perth, Tayside, Scotland.

Acknowledgments

Grateful thanks go to Dr J. C. Scott, Physician Superintendent, Mrs M. Drysdale, Divisional Nursing Officer, and Peter Galliard, Principal Clinical Psychologist, Murray Royal Hospital, Perth, for their support and encouragement throughout the study. Thanks go to the senior management of the hospitals taking part in the study, for their understanding in allowing the survey to take place in their hospitals, and to the psychologists based at these hospitals for the distribution and collection of the research documents. Thanks also go to Mr D. McDonald of the Computer

Department of the University of Dundee for his assistance in the analysis of the data. I am grateful to Miss Ruth Pearson for the typing of the report, and to Blackwell Scientific Publications Ltd for copyright permission. Finally, my thanks go to all nursing staff of the Murray Royal and Murthly Hospitals, Perth; the Royal Dundee Liff Hospital, Dundee; the Sunnyside Royal Hospital, Montrose; and the Lochgilphead Hospital, Argyll and Bute, who gave their assistance to the researcher.

References

Appleby, L., Ellis, N. C., Rogers, G. W. and Zimmerman, W. A. (1961). A psychological contribution to the study of hospital structure. *Journal of Clinical Psychology*, **17**, 390–393.

Jones, R. G. and Galliard, P. (1982). Exploratory study to evaluate staff attitudes towards geriatric-psychiatry. *Journal of Advanced Nursing*, **8**, 47–57.

Miller, A. E. (1978). Evaluation of the care provided for patients with dementia in six hospital wards. Unpublished MSc thesis, University of Manchester.

Miller E. and Gwynne, G. V. (1974). *A Life Apart — A Pilot Study of Residential Institutions for the Physically Handicapped and Young Chronic Sick*. Tavistock Publications, London.

Reznikoff, M. (1963). Attitudes of psychiatric nurses and aides towards psychiatric treatment and hospitals. *Mental Hygiene*, **47**, 354–360.

Savage, B., Widdowson, T., and Wright, T. (1979). Improving the care of the elderly, in D. Towell and C. Harries (Eds), *Innovation in Patient Care*. Croom Helm, London.

Shanley, E. (1981). Attitudes of psychiatric hospital staff towards mental illness. *Journal of Advanced Nursing*, **6**, 199–203.

Towell, D. (1975). *Understanding Psychiatric Nursing*. Royal College of Nursing, London.

Towell, D. and Harries, C. (1979). *Innovation in Patient Care*. Croom Helm, London.

Wells, T. J. (1980). *Problems in Geriatric Nursing Care*. Churchill Livingstone, Edinburgh.

CHAPTER 8

The Development of a Psychiatric Nursing Assessment Form

JOSEPHINE TISSIER

Editor's Comments

Josephine Tissier describes the development and testing of a patient assessment form designed to be used by psychiatric nurses in admission wards as the first stage of systematic care planning. The assessment form should be useful for practice and this Editor, who collaborated in the development of the form, would welcome comments on its usefulness with patients. The study is methodologically interesting as it illustrates some of the complex steps involved in developing and refining any method of patient assessment.

Introduction

This chapter describes the stages undertaken to develop a psychiatric nursing assessment form which is intended to improve and facilitate nurses' collection of information about patients admitted to acute psychiatric wards.

The initial premise underlying this work was that the nursing process model of care, which emphasizes the importance of looking at a patient as an individual and of identifying particular needs before applying nursing interventions, is applicable to the psychiatric setting.

Review of Literature

There has been considerable support from the nursing statutory authorities for the development of the nursing process (Brooking, 1983), and much has been written on this subject (e.g. Jury, 1975; Crow, 1977a;

Marks-Maran, 1979; McFarlane and Castledine, 1982). An awareness of the possible benefits of this system of care in the psychiatric nursing setting has been emerging recently (e.g. Altschul, 1977; Jones, 1980; Keane, 1981; Smyth, 1982). Hills and Wheatley (1981) and Green (1983) implemented the nursing process in their wards, and confirmed its advantages. This, of course, is only anecdotal evidence. An apparent delay, nevertheless, does exist in the implementation of the nursing process in psychiatric nursing and this could be attributable, as Smith (1980) pointed out, to the 'lack of a suitable vehicle for collecting a patient's psychiatric history'.

An essential element in the nursing process, emphasized by several authors (e.g. Marks-Maran, 1979; Darcy, 1982), is that the nurse should collect information in a systematic and continuous manner. To aid the nurse in this task it would seem that a clear and comprehensive form would be invaluable (Schröck, 1980; Cormack, 1980). Two American studies have evaluated the usefulness of a nursing assessment form in practice. In the first study, Hamdi and Hutelmyer (1970) modified an existing assessment tool and examined its effectiveness in the identification of nursing care problems. Ten diabetic patients were assessed by two nurses: one from the experimental group utilizing the tool and one from the control group who did not. Each nurse identified and substantiated nursing problems which were classified as valid or invalid by a panel of three judges. There was no significant difference within the two groups on the number of valid problems identified, but the ratio of valid problems to total problems identified in each group was higher within the experimental group. This group also stated a significantly greater proportion of reasons substantiating the problems.

In the second study, Hefferin and Hunter (1975), examined whether, by introducing onto their general units either an objective observation checklist or a nursing history (*sic*) device into the generally unstructured nursing assessment situation, there would be an increase in the number, scope, clarity, and interrelatedness of care plan entries. The first step was the collection of thirty patient care plans which served as the control group. An observation checklist was then utilized for eight weeks during which time a further thirty care plans were collected. Five months later a nursing history device was introduced and thirty of these histories together with the relevant care plans were collected over the subsequent two months. The introduction of the two forms did not produce any significant change in the scope, clarity, and interrelatedness of care plan entries. There was, however, an increase in the number of identified physical and psychosocial problems and nursing intervention entries, although this increase was only statistically significant for the nursing history device. Although both studies indicated that a structured history form or assessment tool enhanced the nurses' ability to identify patient problems, the results obtained were inconclusive.

A number of nursing assessment/history forms have been designed for use in general and psychiatric settings. Crow (1977b) developed one which she believed could be used for all patients as it allowed for modifications to accommodate different nursing specialties. She tested this form on a few patients, but it seems that no other staff were involved in the testing so it is difficult to evaluate its reliability and validity. McFarlane and Castledine's (1982) nursing history form involves a two-stage assessment; the first stage immediately on admission to provide a baseline for care; the second stage entails a more detailed physical and psychological examination. Their form, although comprehensive, would need to be modified for use in a psychiatric setting. Smith (1980) and Darcy (1982) developed forms specifically for use in psychiatric nursing. Smith (1980) utilized a systems approach, dividing her form into sections each relating to a particular area of a patient's life. However, the psychoanalytic aspect appears to have been omitted. Darcy (1982) emphasized that the nursing history should be established against a background of the 'patients' illness, personality, perception of hospital, and social and family circumstances with particular references to the problems which precipitated hospitalization'. However, the developmental history and sexuality of the patient have been omitted and this could result in an incomplete profile. Snyder and Wilson (1977) developed a tool for psychological assessment and, although not a nursing assessment form, certain aspects of it could usefully be incorporated in one.

In order to derive a theoretical framework for the development of the form several nursing models were examined. Although no conceptual model appears to have been developed as a specific basis for psychiatric nursing practice, elements of existing global nursing models were drawn upon. For example, Roy and Riehl (1974) developed an 'adaptation model' for use in any field of nursing and certain of its concepts were appropriate. However, as Smith (1980) pointed out, Roy's model would be difficult to use in its entirety as the terminology is often ambiguous. Henderson's (1966) model is based on 'activities of daily living'. This focuses largely on patients' physical state, and to subscribe exclusively to it would result in the history form being too physically orientated. Another nursing model advocated by Altschul (1977) for use in the psychiatric setting, is the systems approach. This involves recognition and identification of the systems by which human behaviour is organized, the pressures with which it is designed to cope, and the points at which disorganization and breakdown can occur. This approach is useful as it emphasizes the necessity of exploring the psychiatric patient's motives and behaviour in relation to significant people and events in his life.

There is evidence that psychiatric nurses do not plan care on any theoretical basis of nursing practice, but rather on the prevailing psychiatric ideology in the clinical setting in which they work (Towell, 1975; Schröck, 1980; Cormack, 1983). The most common psychiatric ideologies identified by Schröck (1980) are the biological (somatic, medical), psychological (psychoanalytic), behavioural, and social models. Each model makes different assumptions about the nature of mental disorder, its causes and treatment. Darcy (1982) suggested that nurses need to be aware of these various perspectives. The exclusive use of one model may result in problems being masked by inappropriate interventions.

Keane (1981) stated that the nursing process implies that nurses make assessments of patients' needs. Fulfilment of needs is considered to be essential to an individual's well-being and a deficiency in this sphere could be a contributory factor to the patient's condition. A review of the work of two theorists on this topic, Maslow (1968) and Argyle (1979), was useful, as they provided principles on which the assessment form could be based.

Overall, the literature reviewed not only supported the need for more research in the field but gave some useful indications of the requirements of a psychiatric nursing assessment form.

Research Design

The methods adopted for this study were subdivided into three sections which corresponded to the three main aims: the development of the nursing assessment form; the feasibility testing on the wards; and the effectiveness of the form in aiding nurses to identify nursing problems. It is only possible to reproduce here a summary of the work undertaken and readers requiring further information are referred to the complete research report (Tissier, 1984). At all times throughout the study ethical considerations were borne in mind.

Developing the Nursing Assessment Form

Six phases were carried out in the construction of the assessment form.

Preliminary Exploratory Research

This was undertaken as a guide to format design and to establish areas of information to be included in the form. Firstly, it involved an examination of information collected by third year undergraduate nursing students for their nursing assessments of psychiatric patients. Twenty-six students (including the researcher) had completed a psychiatric nursing course. Each student was required to conduct a nursing assessment and draw up a care plan for one patient during a clinical placement on an acute admission ward. Twenty completed data sheets were examined and a list was compiled of what the students considered as relevant items. These items and other aspects of the format of these sheets were used as a framework for the first draft of the assessment form.

Secondly, interview sessions were held with ward sisters/charge nurses from eight admission psychiatric wards, as well as a consultant psychiatrist, an occupational therapist, a social worker, and a clinical psychologist. Semi-structured interview schedules were used to guide the direction of the interviews but there was plenty of opportunity for free discussion. These interview schedules were designed with the following aims:

1   to determine the current methods of assessment by nurses on the wards and by other members of the multidisciplinary team;
2   to assess the ward sisters'/charge nurses' views on the current methods of assessment and on the need for a structured form;
3   to ascertain the opinions of the members of the multidisciplinary team regarding the role of the psychiatric nurse;
4   to discover the views of all the above staff on the type of information needed for a nursing assessment.

Overall, the staff interviewed felt that a structured assessment form was needed and gave some helpful ideas on its design.

First Draft of the Nursing Assessment Form

This was divided into seven sections:

Section 1   Baseline Admission Information, e.g. name, address, etc.
Section 2   Preliminary Information. This section provided spaces for the nurse to summarize information obtained initially about the patient's emotional, physical and social condition.

It was intended that these two sections should be completed on the first day of admission from information collected through a short interview with patient, relative/friend, and/or a review of existing records/medical notes, and/or nurses' initial observations of the patient.

Section 3   Background Information. This section was designed to elicit the patient's perception of his admission, to define any precipitating events and to record the patient's previous experience of psychiatric hospitals.

Section 4   Physical Health. This covered the basic physical needs.

Section 5   Social/Interpersonal and Developmental Information. This was intended for the nurse to identify social problems in such areas as family, accommodation, work, and any supplementary ones which may have arisen through hospital admission. A review of the patient's developmental history could give a background to the presenting problem and might highlight any past crises.

Section 6   Mental/Emotional Characteristics. This included areas such as self-image, emotions, motivation etc.

The last four sections entailed a thorough assessment, and the information was to be mainly obtained through one or more detailed interviews with the patient, preferably within the first week of admission. The form contained a column of sample questions as an aid for the nurse when interviewing. It also provided space for the nurse to record verbatim or to paraphrase the patient's answers. The degree of formality and the number of interview sessions was left to the judgement of the nurse concerned. Space was provided to record supplementary information from medical notes, friends/relatives, and any other observations. If a patient was unable to respond to a detailed interview within the first week it could be postponed to a more propitious time and the nurse should obtain as much information as possible from supplementary sources.

Section 7   was a single sheet in diagrammatic form for the nurse to summarize the main findings, and could be used for quick reference.

Guidelines for completion of the history form, including hints on interviewing techniques were drawn up.

Validity Testing

The validity of the assessment form rested upon the relevance of the items covered with regard to the form's purpose in psychiatric nursing. The first draft, therefore, was submitted to a panel of fifteen experts in the field of psychiatric nursing and/or nursing process for their comments on format design and content. It is not possible to include here all the many helpful suggestions that were given. The unanimous view, however, was that the form constituted a welcome innovation but was too long and duplicated some of the information collected by medical staff.

Refinement of the First Draft

This was undertaken with the comments of the panel in mind and changes were made in presentation, content, and terminology resulting in a reduction of the form's length by about a quarter.

Testing of the Second Draft

The purpose of this stage was to establish the feasibility of the form, to determine areas for possible revision and clarification and to establish a measure of the reliability of the form. On grounds of expediency and ethics, it was decided to test the form initially on three friends prepared to act as 'pseudo-patients'. This was done by the researcher on each volunteer separately, then by a fellow student immediately afterwards on one of the volunteers. One measure of the feasibility of a form is the amount of time a nurse would need to spend interviewing a patient. The time for interview and completion of this form was approximately one hour.

To determine areas for possible revision and clarification, the pseudo-patients and the fellow student interviewer were asked to comment on the questions, clarity of terms, etc. This threw light on certain areas which needed further refinement.

Inter-rater reliability was examined. Ideally the form should allow for no discrepancies in interpretation so that if different nurses were to use the history form on the same patient, they would be recording similar information. Variables such as expertise in interviewing and rapport with the patient obviously have some bearing on the outcome. In this test for reliability the variables were minimized by choosing a second interviewer equally well known to the pseudo-patient and with similar nursing experience to the researcher, and limiting the time interval between the two interviews. Comparison of the two assessment forms showed that no significant differences in recording information about the same pseudo-patient had occurred and this suggested that there were no ambiguities in the printed content. This was, however, only a subjective measure of reliability.

Final Draft of the Assessment Form

The format of the final draft is shown in the Appendix. A further set of guidelines were drawn up to accompany it and briefly the instructions were as follows:

Stage 1

This should be carried out soon after the patient arrives on the ward. The information is to be gathered by nurses' observations of the patient, a short interview with the patient, relative, or friend, and reference to existing records or medical notes.

Stage 2

This should be completed within the first week of admission. The nurse responsible for the care of the patient is to record observations at the end of every shift.

Stage 3

Towards the end of the first week, and possibly later, the patient should be interviewed once or more. It is emphasized that the nurse should not follow the format of this stage too rigidly and should use discretion as to the most suitable method of obtaining the information. This should be supplemented from interactions with relatives/friends of the patient, and from the findings of other members of the multidisciplinary team.

Stage 4

The summary sheet provides a convenient, concise, and immediate visual record of the patient's profile obtained within the first week of admission. Hints on interviewing techniques were provided to assist nurses.

Assessing the Feasibility of Using the Form on Admission Wards

The final draft of the form was tested on a small sample of patients by the researcher and a group of staff nurses. In both cases the venue for testing was four acute admission psychiatric wards in two hospitals. The criteria that were adopted in the choice of patients were: they should be willing and able to respond to a nursing interview, and be over the age of sixteen. Due to the limited time available, it was only possible for the researcher to interview two patients, both of whom were suffering from depression. They were interviewed within forty-eight hours of admission. Stages 1, 3, and 4 of the nursing assessment form were completed but Stage 2 referring to the nurses' observations of a patient over a period of one week was obviously omitted. The two patients were asked how they had felt about the interview. One stated that normally she disliked talking about herself but that on this occasion she felt able to do so as she knew she would never see the researcher again. The other commented that, 'no nurse (had) gone through my problems in such depth, but I have not liked to trouble the nurses with my problems, they all seem too busy'. This patient felt the interview was helpful as he wanted to talk about his feelings. Subsequently, a comparison was made of the information recorded on the nursing assessment forms with that of the nursing Kardex. In the researcher's view the information obtained was more comprehensive than that entered in the Kardex system.

To give a more accurate picture of the usefulness of the form a sample of four registered mental nurses were each asked to select a patient on whom to complete a nursing assessment form. The four patients chosen represented a cross section of diagnostic categories. The nurses were later interviewed using a semi-structured format. The objectives of the interviews were to identify any problems with the form such as terminology or design, to determine omissions or irrelevancies, to assess ease of use and appropriateness for its intended purpose and to assess its pragmatic validity, i.e. its usefulness.

The main problem identified was the lack of space on the form for nurses to record data. A few minor omissions were also pointed out. All four nurses felt that the form was easy to use and readily understood, but one considered that the work it entailed was too much for one nurse. Another disliked completing a systematic form as he felt it restricted individuality, although he did point out that it would be beneficial for student nurses. It was generally felt that the assessment form would be a useful tool if a greater degree of flexibility were introduced. However, no firm conclusions regarding the form's feasibility can be made unless a larger sample of nurses become involved in its testing and over a longer period of time.

Testing the Effectiveness of the Assessment Form in Aiding Nurses to Identify Nursing Problems

This was based on the hypothesis that a systematic method of collecting and recording patient information would be of greater assistance to the nurse than the current method of documentation (the Kardex system) in identifying nursing problems.

The four assessment forms completed by the staff nurses and the relevant Kardex sheets covering the same time period were collected. The staff nurses had been asked not to record information themselves in the Kardex sheets but to allocate the task to other qualified nurses. To determine the effectiveness of the assessment form in aiding the nurses to identify nursing problems, a random sample of eight fourth year undergraduate nursing students were divided into two groups. The assessment form and Kardex sheets were allocated to them in a 'cross-over' manner (Table 1).

Table 1   Form allocation

Group A

Student no. 1   Given assessment form 1 followed by Kardex 2
Student no. 2   Given assessment form 2 followed by Kardex 1
Student no. 3   Given assessment form 3 followed by Kardex 4
Student no. 4   Given assessment form 4 followed by Kardex 3

Group B

Student no. 5   Given Kardex 2 followed by assessment form 1
Student no. 6   Given Kardex 1 followed by assessment form 2
Student no. 7   Given Kardex 4 followed by assessment form 3
Student no. 8   Given Kardex 3 followed by assessment form 4

This procedure for allocating the forms was adopted to minimize the following extraneous variables:

1   Nurses developing fatigue, boredom, etc. during the task.
2   A carry-over of information that would have resulted if the same student had dealt with the Kardex sheet and assessment form of the same patient.
3   Nurses' differing ability in the task of identifying nursing problems.

The students were asked to list nursing care problems from the information on both of their forms. To obviate the possibility of student bias toward one or other of the forms, they were not given full details regarding the purpose of the exercise. When the students had completed the lists the researcher examined the problems identified to ascertain their validity. Invalid or non-existent problems were disregarded. To increase objectivity, a tutor in psychiatric nursing was asked to do the same task and was given no indication as to whether the problems had come from the Kardex or assessment form. There was a significant increase in the number of problems identified by the student nurses from the information recorded on the assessment forms compared with the Kardex sheets (t-test, $p < 0.1$).

The researcher and her tutor then categorized each of the identified problems as being either physical or psychosocial. All manifestations of a physical nature, although many are probably psychosomatic in origin, were categorized as physical problems. The results are shown in Table 2.

Table 2 Classification of problems identified

Scope	Assessment form	Kardex sheet
Physical	18 (25%)	16 (41%)
Psychosocial	53 (75%)	23 (59%)
Total	71	39

It can be seen from the above table that the increased number of total problems identified from the assessment forms compared to the Kardex sheets was of a psychosocial nature. This was to be expected as the assessment form contained a number of cues in that area, as well as in the physical one. Although it is arbitrary to make a clear division between physical and non-physical problems in the psychiatric setting, it does seem that the assessment form aided the nurses in obtaining a more comprehensive patient profile. This is a positive step which could go some way towards attaining the ideal of 'total' patient care.

Conclusion

The implications of the assessment form for psychiatric nursing were illustrated by the testing of its performance effectiveness. The generally favourable responses given by the staff nurses who tested it on patients admitted to acute psychiatric wards gave evidence of its pragmatic success as a vehicle for gathering information. Furthermore the statistically greater number of nursing problems, with a higher proportion of them being judged as psychosocial, identified by the student nurses from the assessment forms compared to the Kardex sheets, presents a picture which may help to dispel the belief cited by Clarke (1979) that 'all too often the psychiatric nurse has no clear idea of what . . . the patient's problems (are)'.

Unfortunately, due to time constraints, only a limited amount of testing was carried out on the form. The sample numbers throughout were small and no pilot studies were performed. It is possible, too, that researcher bias may have influenced the results. A further criticism might also be voiced that a printed form might be used solely for its own sake, and that the process of recording could become ritualized. A similar reservation was indicated in some of the correspondence that was received from the panel of 'experts'. This form, however, was not developed for use as a rigid checklist or just as an aesthetically pleasing recording system. It was intended to be a tool that could be used systematically, consistently, and concisely to collect information on a patient which would facilitate goal-directed nursing. Furthermore, the form's flexibility allows the nurse to choose the manner and time most convenient to herself and the patient for data collection.

Although the positive results that have been obtained do not testify to the value of the nursing process as a whole in the psychiatric setting, it would seem that the implementation of a nursing assessment form is well worth consideration, not only in acute admission psychiatric wards, but in all psychiatric settings.

References

Altschul, A. T. (1977). Use of the nursing process in psychiatric care. *Nursing Times*, **73**, 1412–1413.

Argyle, M. (1979). *The Psychology of Interpersonal Behaviour*, 3rd edn. Penguin Books, Harmondsworth, Middlesex.

Brooking, J. (1983). The nursing process: report of a seminar. *Nursing Times, Occasional Papers*, **79** (10), 32–34.

Clarke, R. (1979). Assessment in psychiatric hospitals. *Nursing times*, **75**, 590–592.

Cormack, D. F. S. (1980). The nursing process: an application of the S.O.A.P.E. model. *Nursing Times*, **76**, 37–40.

Cormack, D. F. S. (1983) *Psychiatric Nursing Described*. Churchill Livingstone, Edinburgh.

Crow, J. (1977a). The Nursing Process—1. Theoretical background. *Nursing Times*, **73**, 892–896.

Crow, J. (1977b). How and why to take a nursing history. *Nursing Times*, **73**, 950–957.

Darcy, P. T. (1982). *The Process of Mental Health Nursing*. Workbook Publications, Co. Tyrone.

Green, B. (1983). Primary nursing in psychiatry. *Nursing Times*, **79**, 24–28.

Hamdi, M. E. and Hutelmyer, C. M. (1970). A study of the effectiveness of an assessment tool in the identification of nursing care problems. *Nursing Research*, **19** (4), 354–358.

Hefferin, E. A. and Hunter, R. E. (1975). Nursing assessment and care plan statements. *Nursing Research*, **24** (5), 360–366.

Henderson, V. (1966). *The Nature of Nursing*. Collier-Macmillan, London.

Hills, R. and Wheatley, P. (1981). Improving standards in psychiatry. *Nursing Times*, **77**, 2186–2188.

Jones, M. P. (1980). The nursing process in psychiatry. *Nursing Times*, **76**, 1273–1275.

Jury, M. G. (1975). Continuing education for the nursing process skills. *Occupational Health Nursing*, **18**, 18–40.

Keane, P. (1981). The nursing process in a psychiatric context. *Nursing Times*, **77**, 1223–1224.

McFarlane, J. K. and Castledine, G. (1982). *A Guide to the Practice of Nursing using the Nursing Process*. Mosby, London.

Marks-Maran, D. (1979). In the process of better care. *Nursing Mirror*, 12 July, 12.

Maslow, A. M. (1968). *Toward a Psychology of Being*. Van Nostrand, Florence, Kentucky.

Roy, L. C. and Riehl, J. P. (1974). *Conceptual Models for Nursing Practice*. Appleton-Century-Crofts, New York.

Schröck, R. A. (1980). Planning Nursing Care for the mentally ill. *Nursing Times*, **76**, 704–706.

Smith, L. (1980). A nursing history and data sheet. *Nursing Times*, **76** (17), 749–754.

Smyth, T. (1982). Cited in P. T. Darcy (1982), *The Process of Mental Health Nursing*, Workbook Publications. Co. Tyrone.

Snyder, J. C. and Wilson, M. F. (1977). Elements of a psychological assessment. *American Journal of Nursing*, February, 235–239.

Tissier, J. M. (1984). The development and testing of a psychiatric nursing history form. Unpublished dissertation: submitted for the degree of Bachelor of Science to the University of London, Department of Nursing.

Towell, D. (1975). *Understanding Psychiatric Nursing*. A sociological analysis of modern psychiatric nursing. Royal College of Nursing, London.

Appendix
Final Draft of
the Psychiatric Nursing
Assessment Form

Ward . . . .

Stage 1 Baseline Admission Information

. . . . Hospital

Surname:	Patient's date of birth:	Age:	Sex:	Male/Female

First names:
Home address:

Marital status: Date of admission: Time:

Religion: Date of discharge: Time:

Tel no:

Occupation: Section if any:
Next of kin: Date of order: Expiry:
Name: Nationality:
Address:

Hospital number:

Accompanying person:
Name: Care at home:
Address: Social worker:
                                                Tel no:
Tel no: Community nurse:
Relationship with patient: Tel no: Tel no:
Relationship to patient: Health visitor:
                                                Tel no:
Does patient object to relatives   Home help:
being informed?   Yes/No   Family Doctor: Tel no:
(Informal patients only).   Name: Meals on wheels:
Informed of admission?   Yes/No   Address:

Physical observations on admission.   Tel no: Hospital or other place from which
                                                patient is admitted if not home:

Type:	BP	P	T	Urine	Weight	Height

Medications on admission: Tel no:

Result:

Consultant:

Diagnosis: Tick if patient is in receipt of:
                                                (a) Sickness benefit
Known allergies: (b) Pension
                                                (c) Other allowances (specify)
Past medical history, if relevant:

Patient's and family's understanding of condition.

1. Patient's attitude and insight towards admission.

2. Family's attitude towards admission.

3. Patient's perception of family attitude.

Previous experience of psychiatric hospitals.

1. Details of patient's previous admission to hospital, if any.

2. Assess attitude of patient towards previous admission/s and treatment received.

3. Identify any family predisposition to a psychiatric complaint.

General assessment on admission.

Head
- Mental
- Emotional
- Vision/Hearing/Mouth

Trunk
- Respiration
- Circulation
- Temperature
- Skin
- Fluid
- Elimination

Extremities
- Movement
- Sensation

Brief details of patient's physical and emotional state on admission using a systematic head to toe review.

History taken by ....

Stage 2. Murse's Observations and Additional Information from Relatives/Friends and other disciplines

Date	Information required	Data collected
	General appearance and personal hygiene *Note* Patient's motivation to wash, care for clothes etc.; the presence of any psychiatric/physical disabilities impeding or distorting hygiene functioning or causing difficulties with dressing and grooming; the presence of any risk factors in relation to personal hygiene, e.g. suicidal patients during bathing	
	Mood *Note* Patient *appears* depressed, anxious, phobic, elated. Observe facial expression, gestures, etc.	
	Thought Processes and Verbal Behaviour *Note* Presence of hallucinations/delusions/other thought disorders; blocking, vagueness, etc. Specify and describe how patient's behaviour is affected. *Note* Communication difficulties. Any problems due to mental illness, e.g. overtalking/shouting/incoherence/word salads, etc.	
	General attitude *Note* Patient's attitude towards relatives, other patients, staff, e.g. is patient embivalent, sociable, hostile, etc? *Note* Any non-verbal or verbal aggressive behaviour	
	Behaviour and Mannerisms *Note* Obsessional behaviour or rituals, e.g. hand washing. *Note* If patient is restless/overactive/underactive. Consider effects of chemotherapy on movement	

Date	Information required	Data collected
	Orientation and Concentration	
	Note Any confusion. Identify if patient is aware of time/person/place/reality. Assess recent/remote memory	
	Activities of daily living	
	1 Breathing and circulation: *note* any problems e.g. observe for cough, oedema of ankles, skin colour	
	2 Nutrition: *note* any anti-social eating habits. Observe obesity/anorexia	
	3 Fluids: *note* any symptoms of dehydration	
	4 Elimination — Assess presence of rituals/obsessions/delusions in relation to elimination. *Note* any incontinence. Assess how mental illness/drug therapy might affect elimination	
	5 Mobility — Assess patients co-ordination and posture. Consider effects of chemotherapy on movement and posture	
	6 Sleep — Observe if patient has fits/nightmares, etc.	
	7 Senses — Are there risk factors associated with special senses, e.g. vision?	
	8 Medication — *note* any non-compliance	

Stage 3   Detailed assessment

Date	Information required	Date collected
	(A) Patient's attitude towards admission — expectations and goals e.g. Do you feel that you are beginning to settle on the ward? What would you like to achieve from being here in hospital? *Precipitating events of admission — crises/losses/anxiety.* e.g. Has anything been upsetting you lately? (i.e. before admission to hospital). Would you like to tell me about it?	
	(B) Activities of Daily Living 1. *Normal daily schedule* Evaluate ritualistic behaviour and areas of preoccupation. e.g. Can you tell me how you usually spend your day at home? 2. *Sleep and Rest* (a) Establish normal sleeping pattern and any recent problems. e.g. What time do you usually go to bed? How well would you say you normally sleep? Has there been any change recently? Do you have difficulty getting to sleep? Or do you wake early? Do you like to get up in the morning? (b) Assess patient's method of coping with insomnia. e.g. What do you do at home if you can't sleep?	
	3. *Mood — diurnal pattern* e.g. Do you feel better in the morning, afternoon or evening? Do you find your mood changes often? How do you feel most of the time?	

Date	Information required	Data collected
	4. Nutrition (a) Normal dietary habits. Identify any special requirements such as religion, vegetarian, dislikes. e.g. Do you enjoy food? Is there anything that you really cannot eat? Who does the cooking and shopping? (b) Appetite. Identify recent changes. e.g. Has your appetite changed recently? (c) Patient's perception of present appearance. e.g. Are you happy with your present weight?	
	5. Fluids Alcohol. e.g. Do you ever drink alcohol? How often do you drink? How does alcohol affect you? Identify if alcohol is a coping mechanism. e.g. Why do you take alcohol?	
	6. Elimination (a) Establish normal bladder and bowel pattern. e.g. Do you have difficulty passing water? Do you have any difficulties with your bowels? (b) Identify any recent changes. e.g. Have you noticed any change in your bowel or bladder functioning. (c) Assess preoccupation with bowel/bladder functioning. e.g. Do you ever become worried over bowel functioning? (d) Nocturia?	
	7. Physical problems Identify any problems in vision/hearing/smell/touch/taste/speech/walking. e.g. Do you have any problems with sight/hearing/smell/touch/taste? Do you feel unsteady when you are walking? Do you feel you understand what is being said to you? Do you feel other people understand you?	

8. *Comfort and pain*
(a) Identify any presence of pain. e.g. Do you have any aches, pain or headaches, upset stomach?
Do you know if the pain is associated with anything in particular?
(b) Identify normal way of coping with pain. e.g. How do you normally relieve the pain?

9. *Sexuality*
(a) Women. Do you ever feel tense and irritable before a period? How long does the feeling last?
Are your periods painful?
Menopause? Assess reactions.
(b) Sexual orientation. e.g. Are you concerned with sexual relations?
Do you find yourself attracted to men or women?
Do you feel attractive to men or women?
(c) Sexual satisfaction. e.g. Do you find your sex life satisfactory? Are there particular problems or fears you would like to talk about?

10. *Use of chemical agents*
(a) Knowledge of prescribed medication. Compliance/abuse. e.g. Are you taking any tablets? What are they for? Do they seem to help?
(b) Nicotine e.g. How much do you smoke?
Could you give up smoking?
(c) Illicit drugs e.g. Do you ever take drugs that have not been prescribed for you? Why? How do they affect you?
(d) Alcohol. e.g. Do you ever drink alcohol? How often? How does it seem to affect you? Why do you drink?

Date	Information required	Data collected

(C) Social/Interpersonal and developmental information

1. Family History

(a) Childhood. Identify any possible traumatic experiences. e.g. Would you say you had a happy childhood? Can you remember anything which might have upset you which you would like to tell me about?

(b) Identify past relationship with parents (or carers). e.g. What was your relationship like with your parents? Would you say your parents got on well together? Did they row in front of you?

(c) Identify coping mechanisms if problems. e.g. How did you cope with . . . . ?

(d) Identify relationship with siblings as a child. e.g. How did you get on with brothers/sisters? Did you feel an important and loved member of the family? Is there anything about your childhood which you would have liked to have been different?

(e) Identify present relationship with parents/siblings? e.g. Do you still see your parents, brothers, sisters? How do you think they would feel about you being in hospital?

2. Educational History

If still at school/college go on to (c).

(a) Identify emotional response to school. e.g. Did you enjoy being at school? What did you enjoy/dislike at school? How did you feel at school? Did you have a lot of friends?

(b) Identify education achievement and patient's satisfaction. e.g. Were you pleased with your exam results? Were you ever made to feel stupid at school? If patient went to college — identify responses.

(c) If still at school/college identify response. e.g. Do you enjoy school/college? What sort of pressures are you under? Assess relationship with peers. e.g. Have you many friends at school/college? Did you tell them you were coming into hospital? If no — Why not? If yes — how did they react? Identify any problems resulting from admission in terms of education. e.g. How do you feel about taking time off school/college to come into hospital?

3. *Occupation* (If unemployed/retired go on to (c))
(a) Assess satisfaction with job. e.g. Do you enjoy work? Are you under pressures at work that you feel you cannot cope with? Do you feel respected at work?
(b) Identify any problems resulting from admission to hospital in terms of work. e.g. How do you feel about taking time off work to come into hospital? Did you tell your employers/workmates you were coming into hospital? If yes, how did you feel about telling them? If no, why not?
(c) Unemployed or retired. Identify reactions: e.g. How do you feel about not working? What do you do with your time? Was a job a main source of satisfaction in your life?

4. *Marital History*
(a) If single: identify close relationship with own or opposite sex. Any past relationships. Would you say that you have a close relationship with someone? Can you describe the relationship? Have you ever had a relationship? If no, would you like one? How have you coped with break-ups in the past?
(b) If married or living together: identify relationship, e.g. Tell me about your partner. Can you describe your relationship with him/her? Do you find you can talk about problems? Who would you say is the dominant partner? Identify problems. e.g. Have you noticed any difference in your relationship with your partner? Are there any specific difficulties in the relationship which you would like to talk about? Do you find your sex life is satisfactory? Have you any fears or problems?

Date	Information required	Data collected
	(c) If divorced: identify patient's reactions. e.g. How did you feel about splitting up? What helped you get over the divorce? (d) If widowed: identify reactions. e.g. How did you cope with your husband/wife's death? (e) Children: identify parent's relationship with children. e.g. Do you miss your children while you're in hospital? Did you tell your children you were coming into hospital? How did they react? If not, why not?	
	5. Accommodation (a) Identify type. e.g. Do you live in own home/rented/shared/hostel/homeless? (b) Identify any problems. Who do you live with? Have you any problems. e.g. Overcrowding? Are you worried about your place while you are in hospital. e.g. Rent, safety, pets?	
	6. Social situations and leisure activities (a) Assess feelings of isolation. e.g. How do you usually get along with others? In times of stress is there anyone you can turn to? How do you feel in a crowd of people? Do you find it difficult to disagree with people? (b) Leisure: assess ability to become involved and enjoy leisure. Assess use of activity as a coping device. e.g. What sort of hobbies have you got? Do these help you relax and forget tensions, problems etc?	
	7. Religion e.g. Do you have any religious practices that you want to follow while you are in hospital?	
	(D) Mental/Emotional Characteristics 1. Personality (a) Self-image and control of self. e.g. How do you see yourself as a person? What kind of words would you use to describe yourself? Do you like yourself? If you could change yourself, what kind of person would you like to be. (b) Self-respect and control of life situation. e.g. What type of person do others think you are? What do most people think about you? Do you feel in control of your life? What do you do, if things get on top of you (regrets, identity, guilt feelings)?	

e.g. Do you regret anything in your life? Is there something you would rather not have done? What would you say you have accomplished in your life?

2. Emotions

Patient's perception of affective behaviour

(a) Awareness of mechanisms normally used to cope with stress? e.g. Are you ever in a situation where your heart races, and your hands feel sweaty? Do you ever feel nervous? What kinds of things seem to spark this off? How do you cope?

(b) Awareness of feelings of anger/frustration and coping mechanism. e.g. Do you ever feel really angry? What makes you angry? What do you do when you are angry?

(c) Awareness of feelings of destructiveness. Evaluate risk of suicide and violent behaviour. e.g. Do you ever feel like hurting yourself? Do you feel like that now? Do you ever get so angry you could hurt someone else?

(d) Awareness of feelings of fearfulness — paranoid? e.g. Do you feel really afraid? Do you feel got at?

3. Motivation

Identify patient's future goals and hopes. e.g. How do you see the future? Do you feel you have anything to look forward to? If you could make changes in your life, how would you change yourself, your home, your relationship?

Stage 4   Summary Sheet   History taken by . . . .

(A) *Patient's attitude and insight towards admission and any precipitating events:*

(B) *Activities of Daily Living*

(C) *Social/Interpersonal and Developmental Information*

(D) *Mental/Emotional Characteristics*

Any Additional Information

Investigations Type	Arranged	Completed	Results	Nurse's signature
Urine				
Bloods				
X-Ray Skull				
X-Ray Chest				
E.E.G.				
E.C.G.				

CHAPTER 9

Descriptive Study of Chemically Dependent Nurses

MARION TALMADGE REED

Editor's Comments

Marion Reed's chapter is an account of a descriptive study of nurses who were drug addicts and alcoholics attending a weekly therapy group. She used structured interviews to obtain data about the characteristics and history of the twenty-six nurses and the relationship between the addiction and stress.

The problem of chemically dependent nurses is just beginning to appear in this country and is not yet tackled systematically. The American state of Georgia seems to be innovative in developing ways of helping addicted health care professionals. Marion Reed's study provides useful indicators for the development and evaluation of preventive services and treatment programmes in Britain.

Introduction

The problem of chemical dependence in nurses is significant. In the USA, available data show that of 971 disciplinary proceedings involving nurses during the period September 1980 until September 1981, 649 or 67 per cent were related to some form of chemical abuse ('Help for the Helper', 1982). In Britain, the investigating and disciplinary committees of the General Nursing Council of England and Wales annual report 1980–1981 note an increase in the number of cases of misuse of drugs and unprofessional nursing practice (General Nursing Council, 1982).

The reason for concern is two-fold. On a professional level, the danger is that client care will be jeopardized by nurses whose judgment and skills are impaired. On a personal level, it is tragic that nurses suffer untreated while they work among providers of health care services. Research is needed to identify nurses who are at high risk for chemical dependence, to treat those afflicted and thus help the profession to retain valuable nurses.

Theoretical Framework

The theoretical framework for this study was stress theory. Modern man has created a society that subjects human beings to a vast number of stressors, and the effect is often devastating.

Alcohol and other mood changing drugs are a popular choice to deal with overabundant stress. A destructive cycle can be established in which the individual begins to use chemicals to manage stress. The very use of the chemicals increases anxiety (DeRosis, 1979). Drug-free periods become increasingly more anxiety ridden and the individual is faced with problems that are a consequence of the chemical use. It is a short step, in this process, to acquire an addiction to a substance that was initially introduced as a stress relieving measure (DeRosis, 1979).

Nursing, like other health professions, has characteristics that should be regarded as high-risk factors for chemical dependence. The work itself is stressful and demanding. Nurses have a variety of mood-changing drugs available and self-medication is simple. Easy access to drugs tends to be associated with their use (Bissell and Jones, 1981). Changing shifts and unpredictable sleep patterns also contribute to making very tempting the use of alcohol as well as other sedatives and stimulants (Bissell and Jones, 1981). With all the risk factors of nursing it is not surprising that nurses are all too well represented among the populations of those who are chemically dependent.

Purpose of the Study

This study was a descriptive study of a group of nurses who were attending a weekly treatment group for chemically dependent nurses. The purpose was to describe characteristics of chemically dependent nurses and to investigate the relationship of stress to chemical dependence.

The research questions were:

1 What were the characteristics of a group of recovering chemically dependent nurses?
2 In this group of nurses, what was the perceived relationship of stress to the initial use of chemicals?

Definitions of Terms

Characteristic: that which exhibits the distinctive qualities of a person.
Recovering chemically dependent nurses: registered nurses self-defined as chemically dependent and recovering through attendance at a group therapy session.
Stress: non-specific response of the body to any demand made on it, as defined by the subjects.
Chemical/drug: any mind-altering substance, including alcohol.
Initial use: beginning chemical use as defined by subject.

Review of the Literature

The literature review was limited to the problem of chemical dependence within the nursing profession. All studies reviewed were American, as no British studies were found.

Bissell and Jones (1981) studied 100 registered nurses during the early and middle 1970s. All subjects considered themselves alcoholic, were members of Alcoholics Anonymous, and had been abstinent for at least one year prior to the study. The study was conducted via face-to-face interviews.

The subjects were found to be academic high achievers with 66.7 per cent of them having been in the upper one-third of their class. Of the group, 31 per cent reported having attempted suicide, 14 per cent had been arrested and 12 per cent jailed.

The researchers compared the nurses group with a similar sized group of addicted male physicians. The researchers thought it would be more likely that the nurses would be confronted or disciplined by supervisors as compared with the physician group. This turned out not to be true. Many nurses reported voluntarily leaving jobs when they had felt under suspicion and had expected sanctions.

Poplar (1969) studied 90 registered nurses seeking treatment for drug addiction at the National Institute of Mental Health Clinical Research Center. Poplar studied the work of Dr Lyle who had tested nurse addicts from 1960 to 1962, comparing nurse addicts to non-nurse women addicts. Lyle found that addiction in the nurse addicts occurred in adulthood rather than adolescence, drug use was usually solitary, and nurses seldom mainlined. The nurses usually obtained drugs through theft from work, physicians, or forged prescriptions. Poplar administered a questionnaire to the group of 90 nurses. By far, the drug of choice was Demerol (British equivalent Pethidine), followed by morphine, paregoric, codeine, Darvon (Doloxene, nearest UK equivalent) and barbiturates.

Levine *et al.* (1974) studied 12 addicted registered nurses who volunteered for admission to the National Institute for Mental Health Clinical Research Center. All subjects were white women, aged 27–56. They had all had extensive lifelong use of medical services which the researchers believed was directly related to their drug use.

Of the group of 12 nurses, 10 had been in out-patient psychiatric treatment and eight had been hospitalized for psychiatric reasons. The drugs abused were almost exclusively prescription drugs; only one nurse had tried marijuana and none had used hallucinogens, cocaine or heroin. Of the nurses, 42 per cent abused alcohol, 42 per cent abused pentazocine (Talwin), 58 per cent abused meperidine (British equivalent Pethidine), 17 per cent morphine, and 8 per cent hydromorphone.

Jaffe (1982) had discussions with 16 recovering alcoholic nurses, aged 30–45 years. The nurses had an average length of sobriety of 4.5 years. Of the 16, six held a master's degree in nursing and eight had at least one alcoholic parent. The majority of the nurses stated that stress was one of the conditions under which they drank and that they needed to learn alternative patterns of behaviour.

The majority of the studies on chemically dependent nurses were conducted in the 1960s and were done in a highly specialized setting, that of the National Institute of Mental Health Clinical Research Center. This study was designed to augment and update the research and to provide data on subjects from a different background. The studies reviewed also examined nurses who were either alcoholic or drug addicted. This study examined nurses who are chemically dependent and who may have used either alcohol or drugs, or both.

Methodology

In an effort to confront and treat the problem of chemically dependent nurses, nurses in the state of Georgia, USA have formed a programme for impaired nurses, which is modelled on the Disabled Doctors Programme of the Medical Association of Georgia (Talbott *et al.*, 1981). The doctor's programme was begun by Douglass Talbott, MD and is based on a contracted, tightly structured, two-year treatment programme. The programme for impaired nurses has received endorsement from the Georgia Nurses Association and the Georgia Board of Nursing and is helping Georgia to take a leadership role in assisting impaired nurses to return to productive lives.

This study researched nurses who were part of the Georgia programme. The research approach was a descriptive study involving individual face-to-face interviews with the subjects. Little research has been directed toward chemically dependent nurses. Therefore, a descriptive approach allowed the researcher to obtain a diversity of information about this population, and served to provide a foundation for future investigations of chemically dependent nurses. Using an individual interview approach, which is more personal than a distributed questionnaire, decreased the likelihood of non-participation in the study. The individual interview approach also allowed the subjects more flexibility and expression of subjective material.

The researcher developed an interview schedule basing content on suggestions from professionals who have worked with chemically dependent nurses and physicians, on characteristics of other data-gathering instruments described in the literature, and on the theoretical framework. The interview schedule (see Appendix) was divided into nine categories: personal history, family history, educational background, health history, drug history, attempts to cope, consequences of addiction, help-seeking behaviour, and relapse history. The schedule was reviewed by five experts in the field of chemical dependence, including Dr Talbott. The experts reviewed the schedule for appropriateness of content, sequence of the questions, and the impact the interview would have on the nurses.

Permission to conduct the study was obtained from the treatment team of the programme and from the nurses themselves. The population consisted of chemically dependent nurses attending a weekly group therapy meeting. All registered nurses, except those who were in in-patient treatment, were eligible to be in the study. All subjects eligible who were asked to participate did so.

The study was based on the assumptions that subjects gave truthful information during the interviews and were not using chemicals at the time of the interviews. Limitations of the study were that it was not possible to obtain a random sample of chemically dependent nurses. The sample was limited to nurses affiliated with a treatment programme which requires funding or insurance. This factor would exclude nurses from lower socioeconomic classes. Chemically dependent nurses who have achieved sobriety in alternative ways, such as through Alcoholics Anonymous or Narcotics Anonymous exclusively, were not included.

Results of the Study

This section presents the results of the study, statistical tests done on the results, and a discussion of the results. Statistical tests used were either the exact binomial test or the normal approximation to the binomial; significance level was 5 per cent and all tests were two-tailed.

Personal History

Twenty-six subjects were interviewed. All subjects were white. The age range was 23–53 years with a mean age of 35. Of the subjects, five (19 per cent) were male and 21 (81 per cent) were female. Of the total, 12 (46 per cent) were married, four (15 per cent) were divorced, and 10 (39 per cent) had never married.

According to the American Nursing Association's Facts about Nursing (1981), 2 per cent of American nurses are male. Comparing the percentage of men in the sample to the percentage of men in nursing, men were significantly over-represented in the sample. Reasons for this could only be speculated upon. It may be that being male in a primarily female occupation is an added stress that may trigger initial chemical use or it may be that this over-representation reflects higher rates of addiction which have traditionally been found in men.

Significantly fewer of the subjects were married and significantly more had never married when compared with that of the general nursing population. These findings were consistent with relational problems, such as isolation and difficulty in forming meaningful relationships, that many subjects reported.

Family History

Of the subjects, nine (35 per cent) had a parent who was alcohol and/or drug addicted. This was not significantly different from the percentage reported by Jaffe (1982).

It was expected that many of the subjects would have a parent who was chemically dependent and this was supported by the study.

Educational Background

Of the subjects, 88 per cent had diploma or associate degree educational backgrounds, 12 per cent had baccalaureate backgrounds, and none had higher than a baccalaureate degree. Compared to the American Nursing Association (1981) figures, the educational background of the subjects did not differ significantly from the educational background of the general nursing population. It was surprising, however, that no subject had a degree higher than the baccalaureate degree. In the Jaffe (1982) study, six of 16 subjects had a master's degree. It may be that these subjects were younger, or it may be that chemically dependent nurses with higher degrees find working settings with more authority and autonomy and are thus less likely to be confronted.

The subjects were found to be academic high achievers, with 69 per cent having been in the upper one-third of their class. This finding was not significantly different from that reported by Bissell and Jones (1981).

Table 1   Specialty areas of the subjects

Specialty	No.	%
Critical care	11	43
Medical–surgical	3	11
Obstetric	3	11
Operating room	3	11
Psychiatry	2	8
Anesthesiology	1	4
Intravenous therapy	1	4
Pediatrics	1	4
No specialty identified	1	4
Total	26	100

Table 1 summarizes the nursing specialties of the subjects. As described in Table 1, more of the subjects identified their specialty area as critical care than any other area.

This finding suggests that critical care nurses are under particularly severe stress, especially as stressors mentioned by the subjects were severely ill patients.

Health History

Of the subjects, 12 (46 per cent) described their general health as 'excellent' and 14 (54 per cent) described it as 'good'. Regarding psychiatric treatment, nine (38 per cent) reported that they had had psychiatric treatment of some kind. This was significantly fewer than the percentage reported in the Levine et al. (1974) study. This finding is not surprising in that subjects for the Levine study were taken from a highly specialized in-patient psychiatric setting. The subjects in the sample probably more accurately reflect the psychiatric treatment of chemically dependent nurses.

Drug History

Table 2 demonstrates the drugs used by the subjects.

As shown in Table 2, the largest percentage of the subjects used only drugs other than alcohol.

Table 3 outlines drugs of choice reported by the subjects.

Meperidine (Demerol or Pethidine) was the drug of choice reported by most of the subjects (15 or 58 per cent). Alcohol was next (46 per cent) followed by morphine (19 per cent) and marijuana (15 per cent). Both Dilaudid and cocaine were a drug of choice for 12 of the subjects.

Table 2   Drugs used by subjects

Alcohol only	4 (15%)
Drugs other than alcohol only	12 (46%)
Both alcohol and other drugs	10 (39%)

Table 3   Drugs of choice

Drug	No. of subjects	% of subjects
Alcohol	12	46
Narcotics		
Meperidine (Demerol)	15	58
(UK equivalent Pethidine)		
Morphine*	5	19
Hydromorphone (Dilaudid)*	3	12
Tranquilizers		
Meprobamate (Equanil)*	1	4
Diazepam (Valium)*	2	8
Barbiturates		
Tuinal*	1	4
Hypnotics		
Flurazepam (Dalmane)*	1	4
Amphetamines	2	8
Analgesics		
Darvon (UK equivalent Doloxene)	1	4
Pentazocine (Talwin)*	1	4
Antitussive		
Tussionex (no UK equivalent)	1	4
Non-prescription		
Marijuana	4	15
Cocaine	3	12

Note More than one drug of choice was reported by 14 subjects.
*Items known by the same names in the UK and USA.

It appears Demerol remains the drug of choice as reported in 1969 by Poplar as well as in 1974 by Levine et al. Narcotic use has not seemed to vary. Talwin was much less a drug of choice in this study (4 per cent) as compared with the Levine et al. (1974) study (42 per cent). This finding may reflect changing popularity of medications.

The biggest drug difference found in this study was in the use of non-prescription drugs. In the present study four of the subjects reported marijuana as a drug of choice and three reported cocaine. Many more of the subjects had used marijuana, although it was not a drug of choice. Levine et al. (1974) reported none of the subjects had used marijuana or cocaine. This difference probably reflects the changing availability and acceptance of these drugs.

In this study 32 per cent of the subjects reported that their usual route of drug administration was the intravenous route. This finding was very different from the Poplar (1969) study, which reported that nurses seldom mainlined.

There were 15 subjects who were working when they began their drug use. Of these, 10 described their work situation as stressful. Table 4 outlines sources of stress identified by the subjects.

The sources of stress identified by the subjects were similar to those described in the literature. Although little can be done about severely ill patients, if nursing recognizes this as a stressor, peer group support and mental health nurse consultation may reduce the stress. Inadequate staffing and shift changes are also difficult problems to deal with. Again, it is important that they be recognized as sources of stress. The unrealistic expectations that nurses have of themselves, with resulting feelings of inadequacy, also need to be recognized as a major source of stress.

Most of the subjects (64 per cent) obtained their drugs through theft from their workplace. This finding has implications for more careful scrutiny of drug records as well as education to teach supervisors what to look out for when theft is suspected. Catching nurses earlier would not

Table 4   Sources of stress identified by subjects

Source of stress	% of subjects reporting
Severely ill patients	60
Understaffing	60
Feelings of inadequacy	50
Problems with shift changes	30

Note   Subjects reported more than one source of stress.

Table 5   Complications of chemical dependence

Complication	Number	Percentage
Automobile accidents	11	42
Arrests	10	38
Suicide attempts	4	15
Jailings	3	12

solve the problem, but would protect patients as well as perhaps getting nurses into treatment earlier.

Table 5 outlines consequences of chemical dependence.

As shown in Table 5, 38 per cent of the subjects had been arrested, which is significantly more than reported in the Bissell and Jones (1981) study. This relates to the fact that these subjects had arrests related to theft of narcotics, while the Bissell and Jones study was of alcoholic nurses.

Attempts to Cope

Of the subjects, seven (27 per cent) had changed work hours to time of less supervision, such as the night shift, and nine (35 per cent) had either quit a job or been fired because of drug use.

Consequences of Addiction

A surprising 25 (96 per cent) of the subjects reported that they had no difficulty in getting jobs, even when their previous employers had suspected them of drug use. Licensure difficulties were reported by 13 (50 per cent) of the subjects and 21 (81 per cent) had relational difficulties, such as family problems and lack of closeness.

Many subjects believed that the lack of difficulty in getting employment was related to the critical shortage of nurses, as their references were sometimes not checked at all.

Significantly more of the subjects had licensure difficulties than in the Bissell and Jones study, again due to differences in populations. Licensure difficulties in the present study were related mostly to theft of narcotics and resulting sanctions from licensing boards.

Table 6 sums up comparisons of subjects to other studies.

Help-seeking Behaviour

Most (88 per cent) of the subjects could identify a precipitating factor for their seeking help. Of this 88 per cent, 35 per cent said the factor was

Table 6   Comparison of subjects to other findings

Variable	Source of comparison	Current findings
Sex (% male)	*A.N.A. (1981)	Over-representation
Marital status	A.N.A.	Fewer married
Psychiatric hospitalization	Levine *et al.* (1974)	Fewer hospitalized
Out-patient psychiatric treatment	Levine *et al.*	Fewer had psychiatric treatment
% Arrested	Bissell and Jones (1981)	More arrested
Licensure difficulties	Bissell and Jones (1981)	More with licensure difficulties
Divorce rate	A.N.A.	N.D.†
Alcohol/drug addicted parent	Jaffe study (1982)	N.D.
Educational background	A.N.A.	N.D.
Academic ranking	Bissell and Jones (1981)	N.D.
Quit job or fired	Bissell and Jones (1981)	N.D.
Suicide attempts	Bissell and Jones (1981)	N.D.
Jailings	Bissell and Jones (1981)	N.D.
Times of unemployment	Bissell and Jones (1981)	N.D.

*A.N.A.:   American Nursing Association.
†N.D.:   No difference.

either the threat of loss of their nursing licence or its actual loss. This suggests that the profession of nursing can be very influential in getting nurses to treatment through appropriate confrontation and threat of licence loss.

Relapse History

Of the subjects, eight had experienced a relapse. Of these eight, seven could identify a precipitating factor, all involving stress. This finding has implications both for treatment teams and for those nurses about to enter a stressful time.

Conclusion

At the end of the interview subjects were asked what they would like the profession of nursing to know about chemical dependence. Of the subjects, 17 (65 per cent) stressed the need for education about chemical dependence, nine (35 per cent) shared the belief that there is 'help and hope' and five (19 per cent) warned that chemical dependence is a very easy pattern for nurses to slip into.

The subjects overwhelmingly emphasized the need for education about the incidence and course of chemical dependence. Many said that nurses need to know it is not a moral issue, but a treatable illness. Subjects felt nurses need to be educated about the incidence of the illness in their own profession and need to learn to support and help one another. Many felt that peers and supervisors knew what was happening to them, but did nothing. They spoke of the guilt and shame they had experienced and stated that the chemically dependent nurse needs treatment not condemnation. They also gave a message of hope. As one subject summed up, 'The only wrong thing to do is to do nothing for the chemically dependent nurse'.

Conclusions of the Study

Based on the data and findings, the following conclusions seem warranted:

1   Male nurses and critical care nurses are at higher risk for chemical dependence than are other nurses.
2   Chemically dependent nurses are likely to have a parent who is chemically dependent.
3   Chemically dependent nurses do not differ from the general nursing population in the percentage of graduates from baccalaureate, associate degree, and diploma backgrounds.
4   Chemically dependent nurses are academic high achievers.
5   The drug of choice remains Demerol (Pethidine).
6   Cocaine and marijuana are frequently drugs of choice.
7   Nurses commonly use the intravenous route.
8   Drug use is solitary.
9   Nurses usually obtain drugs through theft from their workplace.
10 Stress is an important factor both in beginning drug use and in relapse.
11 Even when experiencing the consequences of their illness, most chemically dependent nurses have no trouble obtaining employment.
12 Messages from the nurses themselves concern the need for education about chemical dependence, the need to confront and treat nurses early, the belief that there is 'help and hope' for chemically dependent nurses, and the firm conviction that nurses need to take care of themselves as well as others.

Recommendations for Further Research

Based on the data and conclusions, the researcher offers the following recommendations for further research:

1 Replication of this study in other states and countries to determine whether characteristics in this study are unique or are part of a national and international trend.
2 Replication of this study with nurses who obtained sobriety solely through self-help groups to see if and how they differ.
3 Follow-up studies on this sample to determine the efficacy of the treatment programme. This would be especially powerful if results could be compared to a sample of nurses who attended self-help groups only.

Recommendations for Nursing Practice

Based on the data and conclusions, the researcher offers the following recommendations for nursing practice.

1 Education is necessary for nursing students, practising nurses, and administrators, to inform them of the incidence of the problem in nursing, about the course and symptoms of chemical dependence, and behavioural clues to its presence.
2 Confrontation skills to confront the chemically dependent nurse need to be taught.
3 Professional nursing associations, as well as licensing boards, in working with treatment centres, need to use their powerful intervention tool, the licence, to get chemically dependent nurses to treatment.
4 Tighter monitoring of controlled substances seems indicated, based on the ease with which nurses obtained drugs.
5 Stress management for all nurses, but especially male nurses and critical care nurses, is indicated. Stress management may take the form of group support and mental health nurse consultation. It seems that unless we, as nurses, learn to deal with stress, we are in a vulnerable position to get caught in the destructive pattern of chemical dependence.

Acknowledgments

The author would like to express gratitude to Carol Bush and Rose Dilday of Emory University, Atlanta for their guidance, support, and enthusiasm.

A very special note of thanks is due to the nurses themselves who made the research possible and did so with the kind giving of their time as well as the often painful revelations of their personal histories, with the hope that their stories would help suffering colleagues.

References

American Nursing Association (1981). *Facts About Nursing 1980–1981*. AJN Co., New York.
Bissell, L. and Jones, R. (1981). The alcoholic nurse. *Nursing Outlook*, February, 96–101.
DeRosis, H. A. (1979). *Women and Anxiety*. Delacorte Press, New York.
General Nursing Council of England and Wales (1982). *Professional Discipline*. General Nursing Council, London.
Help for the helper (1982). *American Journal of Nursing*, **82**, 578.
Jaffe, S. (1982). Firsthand views of recovery. *American Journal of Nursing*, **82**, 578–579.
Levine, D., Preston, S., and Lipscomb, S. (1974). A historical approach to understanding drug abuse among nurses. *American Journal of Psychiatry*, **131**, 1036–1037.
Poplar, J. (1969). Characteristics of nurse addicts. *American Journal of Nursing*, **69**, 117–119.
Talbott, G. D., Richardson, A. C., Mashburn, J. S., and Benson, E. B. (1981). The Medical Association of Georgia's disabled doctors program: A 5-year review. *Journal of the Medical Association of Georgia*, **70**, 545–549.

Appendix

Interview Schedule

Personal History

1 What is your age? 20–25____ 26–30____ 31–35____ 36–40____
   41–45____ 46–50____ 51–55____ 56–60____ over 60____
2 Ethnic background: White____ Black____ Oriental____ Hispanic____
3 Are you: the oldest child____ middle child____ youngest____
   only child____ other____ ?
4 Sex: Male____ Female____
5 Are you married? Yes____ No____
   If no: never married____ divorced____ widowed____ separated____
6 Do you have children? Yes____ No____
   If yes, how many?____
        age range____

Family History

7 Are either of your parents alcohol- and/or drug-addicted?
   Yes____ No____ Not sure____
   If yes, which parent? Mother____ Father____
8 Do you have any relatives other than parents who are addicted?
   Yes____ No____
   If yes, who is it? Sibling____ Grandparent____ Child____ Other____

Educational Background

9 What type of nursing program did you attend?
   Diploma____ A.D.____ B.S.____ Graduate____ Doctoral____
10 What year did you graduate?
11 In your professional school(s), did you rank: in highest ⅓ of class____
   in middle ⅓ of class____ in lowest ⅓ of class?____
12 Do you have other credentials, such as:
   A.N.A. certification____ other professional certification? _____
   _____
13 Are you working?____
14 What is your nursing speciality? med/surg____ ob/gyn____
   child health____ critical care____ psychiatry____ nurse anaesthetist____
   other _____
   none specified____

Health History

15 Have you ever had surgery? Yes____ No____
   If yes, list dates and names of operations.
16 Do you have any chronic health problems, such as allergies, diabetes,
   asthma? Yes____ No____ If yes, what are they?
17 How would you describe your general health? Excellent____ Good____
   Fair____ Poor____
18 Have you ever had psychiatric treatment? Yes____ No____
   If yes, was it: in-patient____ (how many times?____) out-patient____
   What is your psychiatric diagnosis? _____
   _____
   Are you presently in psychiatric treatment?____

Drug History

19 What were your drugs of choice?
20 When you initially began using drugs, was it:
   a prescription____ self-treatment____ experiment____ other? _____
   _____
21 When you began using drugs, were you: a
   student____ working____ other? _____
   _____

If working, was the environment that of: ICU____ ER____ OR____
staff nurse____ clinic____ community agency____ other? _____
Would you say your work environment at the time you initially began
using drugs was particularly stressful? Yes____ No____
If yes, what were the stressors?

22 How did you usually obtain your drugs? prescription____
    forging prescription____ theft from workplace____ street drugs____
    other _____

23 What was your usual pattern of using drugs? alone____ with others____

24 Did you usually take the drug: p.o.____ i.v.____ other? _____

25 Are you an alcoholic? Yes____ No____
    If yes, at what age did you begin drinking? _____
    When you began drinking, was it: social drinking____ to relax?____
    Did you usually drink: alone____ with others?____

26 Have you ever been arrested? Yes____ No____
    If yes, please list charges.

27 Have you ever been jailed? Yes____ No____
    If yes, what were the charges?

28 Have you had automobile accidents? Yes____ No____ If yes, how
    many?

29 Have you ever attempted suicide? Yes____ No____ If yes, how?
    If yes, did it occur while you were under the influence of alcohol/drugs?
    Yes____ No____

Attempts To Cope

30 Did you ever change your work hours to time of less supervision, such
    as the night shift? Yes____ No____

31 Did you ever quit a job because you felt you were under suspicion?
    Yes____ No____

Consequences Of Addiction

32 Have you had times of unemployment because of your addiction?
    Yes____ No____ If yes, was this because of: getting fired____
    your choice____ too ill physically____ other? _____

33 Did you have difficulty getting jobs? Yes____ No____
    If yes, please describe:

34 Are you having licensure difficulties? Yes____ No____
    If yes, has your license been: suspended____ probated without limits____
    probated with limits____ revoked____ other? _____

35 Have you had problems with important relationships in your life because
    of your addiction? Yes____ No____
    If yes, what were they?

Help-Seeking Behaviour

36 From whom did you first seek help for your addiction? Psychiatrist____
    Non-psychiatric M.D.____ Clergy____ Nurse____ Impaired Health

Professional____ Family____ Friends____ A.A.____ N.A.____
Other _____

37 What was the precipitating factor? Threat of licence loss____
licence loss____ threat of loss of important person____ loss of important
person____ other_____

38 What phase of the Impaired Nurse Programme are you in? phase I
(in-patient)____ phase II (out-patient)____ phase III (after-care)____
(How long in phase III?____) Finished Impaired Nurse Programme____
(How long finished? _____)

39 How did you hear of the Impaired Nurse Programme? from a nurse in
the programme____ from another nurse____ from a physician____ from
GNA publicity____ other _____

Relapse History

40 Have you ever had a relapse? Yes____ No____
If yes, how many: one____ more than one____ (state number)
What was the precipitating event(s)? _____
_____

What helped you back to treatment? _____
_____

41 What are your goals for the future? To regain licence____ To regain
job____ Other _____

42 Is there anything else you think it would be helpful for me to know?

*Part D   Behavioural Psychotherapy by
Psychiatric Nurses*

CHAPTER 10

National Follow-up Survey
of Practising Nurse Therapists

CHARLES BROOKER and
MARTIN BROWN

Editor's Comments

Charles Brooker and Martin Brown describe in this chapter their national
survey of practising nurse behaviour therapists who have undertaken a
statutory clinical course in Adult Behavioural Psychotherapy. The results
provide a clear picture of their personal and professional profiles, methods
of work organization, and career aspirations.

The authors draw attention to many of the problems experienced by
this group of nurses, who are described as being at a crossroads in their
development. The paper provides vital information upon which to plan
further developments in this aspect of nursing and raises many additional
research questions.

Introduction

This study is about a group of nurses who have undertaken an
advanced clinical training in psychiatric nursing. The subjects, all
Registered Mental Nurses, have successfully completed the Joint Board
of Clinical Nursing Studies course number 650 (now an English National
Board Clinical Course) in Adult Behavioural Psychotherapy. Graduates
of this course have been identified in the literature by various titles
including nurse behaviour psychotherapists or more commonly nurse
therapists.

The aims of this study were to establish:

1 the personal and professional profiles of trained nurse therapists;

177

2   the way in which nurse therapists organize their work after training;
3   the career aspirations of nurse therapists.

In order to understand more fully the aims of the present study, it is
necessary to examine briefly the evolution of nurse therapy training. Bird
et al. (1979) identified the major historical pressures which led to the
establishment of the first nurse therapy training programme. These were
seen as a need to establish effective economic community-based psychiatric
services coupled with a general desire on the part of nurses to develop
their clinical role. In 1972 the Department of Health and Social Security
agreed to fund a three-year experimental research programme that
examined the effectiveness of nurses as the main therapist for a selected
group of adult neurotics. This led to the formal approval by the JBCNS
of an 18-month course in adult behavioural psychotherapy. The first course
commenced in 1975 at the Maudsley Hospital with Professor I. Marks,
a psychiatrist, as course director. Subsequently, courses were established
at Graylingwell Hospital, Chichester, and Moorhaven Hospital, Plymouth,
under the direction of psychologists.

   Nurse therapy research has largely focused on the clinical outcome of
clients treated during training (Marks *et al.*, 1977; Marks *et al.*, 1978).
Nurse therapists have published in a similar vein, mostly describing the
outcome of single cases (Brown, 1980; Brooker, 1980; Sawyer, 1983;
Millar, 1977). While the evidence is indisputable that nurse therapy trainees
are effective for clients, and indeed the training is envied by other
professions (Hall, 1979), as yet little detailed research has been conducted
into the effect of nurse therapy training and practice on the nurses
themselves. Hence this study looks at the ways in which nurse therapists
work after completing training, their career aspirations, and the perceived
benefit of undertaking the course. As the training programmes are now
well established and expanding, it is vitally important for the nursing
profession to address these issues.

Method

The Sample

The sample consisted of every nurse who had completed the Joint Board
of Clinical Nursing Studies course number 650 at the three national training
centres (Maudsley, Graylingwell, and Moorhaven Hospitals), by 1 June
1983. A decision was made not to administer questionnaires to those

Table 1   The eligibility of the total sample

	n	%
Final selected sample	66	88.0
Emigrated	6	8.0
Left nursing	1	1.3
Not in full-time employment	2	2.7
Total no. of trained nurse therapists (June 1983)	75	100.0

trained nurse therapists who were known to have emigrated, left nursing altogether or were no longer in full-time nursing employment. This information was obtained from the National Nurse Therapist Register located at the Maudsley Hospital training centre. We are grateful to Messrs E. Millar, F. McAffrey, and P. Lindley who compiled this register from 1978 to 1983. The exclusion of the nine trained nurse therapists outlined in Table 1, allowed us to direct the survey to all trained nurse therapists currently in full-time employment as psychiatric nurses. That some 88 per cent of trained therapists were eligible, using this criterion raises issues that will be highlighted in the discussion.

Survey Method

The aims of any survey and the kind of data it seeks to obtain should influence the method employed in ideal circumstances. This research, however, was severely restricted by financial constraints. The idea of personally interviewing the sample, although an attractive strategy, was discarded. The costs involved in interviewing such a small, geographically scattered group were too prohibitive.

Postal surveys are comparatively less expensive and this approach was adopted in the light of both the well-reported advantages and disadvantages of this method (Moser and Kalton, 1979; Hoinville and Jowell *et al.*, 1978; Erdos, 1970). The major problem when sending a questionnaire through the post is non-response, which can lead to significant biases in survey results. Unless a survey researcher corrects his results for non-responders, the assumption made is that responders and non-responders are alike in all respects. There is a growing body of experimental research which suggests that this is not the case (Dunkelberg and Day, 1973; Daniel, 1975). When a postal survey method is employed, the aim is to maximize response, thereby reducing non-response bias. In this survey, the following strategies were adopted: a stamped, addressed envelope was enclosed with the questionnaire; a covering letter outlining the survey's aims was included; a reminder letter was sent 3 weeks after first mailing; and finally, 4 weeks after the initial mailing, personal contact was made with non-responders at a Royal College of Nursing–Psychiatric Society Behaviour Therapy Forum Annual General Meeting.

Postal surveys are an appropriate tool for research when the survey aims are clear and when the questions asked are concise and unambiguous. Moser and Kalton (1979) state:

> A mail questionnaire is most suited to surveys whose purpose is clear enough to be explained in a few paragraphs of print; in which the scheme of questions is not over-elaborate; and in which the questions require straightforward and brief answers. (p.260)

The second attraction of mail surveys is the manner in which they reduce response error. Personal interviews, however well planned, are prone to interviewer effects (or variability) which can lead to significant reductions in the validity and reliability of the survey results (Brooker and Wiggins, 1983; O'Muirchearraigh and Wiggins, 1981). Thus a considerable advantage of mail surveys is the increase in the precision of the survey results through the loss of interview variability.

Questionnaire Design

Two main factors decided the design of the questionnaire: the aims of the survey, as outlined earlier, and the use of the postal survey method. It was important that questionnaire design was attractive, easy to fill in, undemanding, and instructions were easy to follow. Otherwise, the response rate would be low. Accordingly, the questionnaire content was arranged to maximize cooperation. This involved asking several questions that would be of high interest to all respondents, because they were directed at the respondents' opinions rather than being merely descriptive of behaviour and characteristics.

The questionnaire was redrafted four or five times and piloted with the current group of nurse therapist trainees ($n = 9$) at the Maudsley Centre. This proved a useful exercise for several reasons. Firstly, the trainees were quick to point out questions that they felt were either ambiguously worded or unnecessarily complex. Secondly, the researchers were able to estimate that, on average, the questionnaire took only 20 minutes to complete. This information was subsequently offered as an inducement to the respondents in the introductory letter. Furthermore, several of the comments elicited from the trainees in the pilot phase indicated that they would have felt more able to give 'open' information if they had been assured that their answers were anonymous. Subsequently, this option was given to all respondents in the main survey.

Response Rate

The nurse therapist survey obtained a response rate of 77.3 per cent ($n = 66$) which varied from 70 to 87 per cent according to training centre, as Table 2 demonstrates. It is tempting to explain the high response rate from Maudsley-trained nurse therapists by the fact that both authors trained at this centre.

Table 2 Response rate by training centre

	%	n
Maudsley	87	33
Graylingwell	79	11
Moorhaven	70	7
Data not valid	6	4
Non-responders	16.7	11
Total	100.0	66

Methods of Analysis

The data were analysed using the BREAKDOWN, CROSSTABS, and ANOVA Sub-Programmes on the Statistical Package For The Social Sciences Computer Programme (Nie *et al.*, 1970). Two basic statistical tests of significance were used: Analysis of Variance (ANOVA) and Chi-Square.

Results

Personal and Professional Profile of Trained Nurse Therapists

The sample consisted of 77 per cent of all eligible trained nurse therapists who completed and returned the postal questionnaire. All respondents were currently working in various types of clinical setting. The mean age of the sample was 33.2 years (range 25 to 48) and males outnumbered females by a ratio of approximately 2:1. A breakdown of the respondents by marital status revealed that 83 per cent were married.

The clinical experience following basic training of the sample ranged from 3 to 25 years (mean 8.2 years). In addition to being on the register for the mentally ill, 33 per cent of the respondents were also State Registered Nurses. Twenty per cent of trained nurse therapists have obtained additional academic and nursing qualifications since completing JBCNS course number 650. These include Social Science and Psychology degrees and Clinical Teacher and Nurse Tutor certificates.

On average, all graduates from JBCNS course number 650 have been working as nurse therapists for 3.5 years, although, of course, this varies from 6 months to 8 years. A small proportion (21.6 per cent) of nurse therapist trainees are seconded to the training course by their employing authority. The largest percentage (78.4 per cent) are funded directly from the individual course centres' training budgets. The small numbers seconded may be because the course is the longest (18 months) approved by the English National Board.

Current Organization of Work

Table 3 identifies the titles which nurses therapists use to describe themselves at work. As suggested in the introduction, the most common title used is 'Nurse Therapist', although nearly 40 per cent of the sample call themselves something different. In total, 70.5 per cent of trained nurse therapists have titles which suggest they work predominantly as clinicians.

Table 4 shows information that relates to nurse therapists' current pay grades. In total, 76.5 per cent of the sample are being paid at one or other of the sister/charge nurses grades. A large number (approximately 60 per

Table 3   Titles used by nurse therapists

Title	%	n
Community psychiatric nurse	8.2	4
Nurse therapist	65.3	32
Nurse teacher	12.2	6
Nurse manager	8.2	4
Research worker	6.1	3
Total	100.0*	49*

*This entry was incomplete for two questionnaires.

Table 4   Nurse therapists' current pay grades

Pay grade	%	n
Sister/charge nurse (2)	47.1	24
Sister/charge nurse (1)	29.4	15
Nursing officer (1)	9.8	5
Clinical teacher	9.8	5
Nurse tutor	3.9	2
Total	100.0	51

Table 5   Nurse therapists' work bases

	%	n
Psychology department	13.7	7
Community psychiatric nursing department	25.5	13
Behaviour therapy unit	17.6	9
Day hospital	3.9	2
Ward	3.9	2
Psychiatric unit	11.6	6
Other	23.5	12
Total	100.0	51

cent) of JBCNS course number 650 trainees were being paid at this level prior to training.

Overall, 73 per cent of the money to pay nurse therapists comes from nursing service budgets, with an additional 16 per cent of posts funded by either nurse education or management budgets. In one instance, finance for nurse therapy posts has come from a general practice in conjunction with the local family practitioner committee, and in another case from a regional health authority.

Nurse therapists use a wide variety of settings for a work base as Table 5 demonstrates. It is an interesting finding that most nurse therapists are attached to community psychiatric nursing departments. Other less common bases for nurse therapists include psychology departments, day hospitals, wards, psychotherapy units, and general practices.

Table 6 shows the results that were obtained when nurse therapists were asked to estimate the percentage of referrals received from all possible sources. Wide variations in working practice are revealed by these data. For example, some nurse therapists received none of their referrals from psychiatrists while others received 99 per cent. One explanation for this result may be the different emphasis of the various training programmes. Moorhaven-trained nurse therapists take significantly more referrals from general practitioners than therapists from either of the other two centres (on average around 52.0 per cent). Correspondingly, Maudsley-trained nurse therapists take more referrals from psychiatrists. As Table 6 shows, general practitioners and psychiatrists are the two largest sources of referral. It is interesting to note that one nurse therapist receives 62 per cent of referrals from community psychiatric nurses.

Eighty-five per cent of trained nurse therapists are still actively maintaining a caseload. Table 7 shows that at any one time there is an average of 25.7 clients on nurse therapists' caseloads. Further, nurse therapists see a mean of 6.8 new cases a month, and on average each nurse therapist discharged 45.8 clients in 1982. This type of 'caseload activity' data would be interesting to compare with community psychiatric nurses, especially those nurse therapists working in community psychiatric nursing teams.

None of the wide variation in caseload activity is explained by differences in training centres, as were the variations in referral source.

The sample of nurse therapists surveyed estimated that the greatest proportion of their time was spent in clinical work (on average 16 hours

Table 6   Percentage of referrals by referral source

Referral source	Average* (%)	Range (%)
Psychiatrist	43.0	0–99
Psychologist	6.0	0–56
General practitioners	29.0	0–96
Social workers	5.0	0–90
Others	17.0	0–62
Total	100.0	

*The figures in this column are expressed as an average percentage for the total sample.

Table 7   Nurse therapists' caseload activity

NT's caseload activity	Mean no.	Range	n
New cases (monthly)	6.8	1–30	41
No. on current caseload	25.7	3–60	41
Discharges (1982)	45.8	10–170	32

per week), the rest of their nursing activity involved liaison with other professionals (3.75 hours), record keeping (4 hours), teaching (4.5 hours), administration (4.5 hours), and research (3 hours). As so much of a nurse therapist's time involves clinical work, it seemed pertinent to ask where clinical supervision was sought and Table 8 presents these results.

The results show that 82 per cent of trained nurse therapists say that no-one actually supervises their clinical work. This finding will be elaborated upon more fully in the discussion.

Table 8   Supervision of clinical work

Supervisor	%	n
Nurse	8.0	4
Psychologist	2.0	1
Doctor	6.0	3
No-one	82.0	41
Other	2.0	1
Total	100.0*	50*

*One response uncodeable.

Current Job Satisfaction and Joint Board of Clinical Nursing Studies Course Number 650

The questions in this section were specifically designed to ascertain the attitudes of trained nurse therapists to the course itself, whether it had been worthwhile, and how it would ultimately benefit the respondents' professional development as nurses.

A total of 86 per cent of the nurse therapists felt that taking the course had been 'essential' to them and, furthermore, 75 per cent felt that it would ultimately benefit their careers. The following are typical of the comments that were made:

'The training made my clinical skills more competent and this increased my confidence.'

'I feel much better prepared professionally and more effective clinically. I developed on a personal level too.'

However, 25 per cent of the sample felt that JBCNS, course number 650 had not benefited their careers. This group made the following kinds of comments:

'I have become disillusioned with the lack of career prospects and bored with clinical work.'

'Unless I am careful and lucky, I shall not be upgraded further.'

'The course has not benefited my career in terms of career prospects, I feel we have specialized up a cul-de-sac.'

Perhaps the strongest remarks were made by one respondent who has actually left nursing to pursue five years of training to become a clinical psychologist:

'I was dissatisfied with endless years of talk about a clinical career structure and zero action and the continued expression of nursing to be a profession is in frequent contrast to its behaviour in many respects. A profession which can select, train and give qualifications to well motivated, highly competent, clinical nurses and then fail wholly to provide an appropriate framework for them to work in seems muddled, directionless and short-sighted. One wonders how much longer 650 (*sic*) trainees will live in hope.

To conclude then, this survey has produced results which may seem slightly paradoxical. Very few of the nurse therapists have left nurse therapy although most of them receive salaries similar to those received before they took the course. They are mature clinical nurses practising advanced clinical skills for little reward. Yet most of them see the training they received as essential, are likely to be employed in the same job in three years time, and feel that being a nurse therapist will ultimately benefit their career.

Discussion

As well as specific aims outlined in the introduction to this study, it was hoped to discover to what extent nurse therapists were integrated in the mainstream of psychiatric nursing as a whole. It was not our aim to compare individual styles and methods of practice. The study was intended to be purely descriptive and, in some senses, this limits the conclusions we can draw. However, it is hoped that this research may help to focus nurse therapists' attention on their relationship with other psychiatric nurses, especially given the need for a clinical career structure in psychiatric nursing.

Personal and Professional Characteristics

There are broad similarities in the personal and professional characteristics of nurse therapists when compared with graduates of all other JBCNS psychiatric course takers (see Table 9, source: Rogers, 1983).

The preponderance of men in nurse therapy has been noted before (Bird *et al.*, 1979) and this study confirms a continuation of the trend. However, as Table 10 suggests, the overwhelming number of men is not solely a trend in nurse therapy but one that extends to all takers of post-basic courses in psychiatric nursing. Men number some 25 per cent of all psychiatric nurses, yet this small group constitute some 66 per cent of post-basic course entrants.

A tentative explanation for these findings is that males perceive the benefit of post-basic education to be related to career progression. It may well be that men take all JBCNS courses in the belief that clinical specialization leads to upward mobility in career path. In a major survey undertaken by Rogers (1983) of all joint board course attenders, psychiatric

Table 9   A comparison of the characteristics of all JBCNS psychiatric course graduates with nurse therapist course graduates

	Nurse therapist (source: survey results)	All other JBCNS psychiatric course graduates (source: Rogers, 1983)
Age	33.2 (mean)	No data
Married	83% ($n = 42$)	71% ($n = 107$)
SRN and RMN	33% ($n = 17$)	35% ($n = 53$)
RMN only	48% ($n = 25$)	42% ($n = 49$)

Table 10   A comparison of male and female sex ratios in psychiatric nursing

	Sex ratio Male : Female
All psychiatric nurses (Source: HMSO, 1982)	1 : 3
Nurse therapists (Source: survey results)	2 : 1
All other post-basic psychiatric course takers (Source: Rogers, 1983)	1.8 : 1

nurses identified the major benefit of post-basic education as the fact that
the qualification led to future promotion. Rogers further summarized
men's motives in the following way:

'The present study has demonstrated that male nurses who
complete post-basic clinical courses are likely to aim for senior
posts in nursing. (p. 239)

The findings of this survey, however, would tend to suggest that
undertaking the nurse therapist course rather than enhancing career
prospects, tend to diminish them. This, of course, is a problem not only
for nurse therapists but for almost all other clinical nurse specialists.

Work Organization

Referral Sources

Table 11 demonstrates clearly the variation in referral agencies which nurse
therapists use, on completion of training. Perhaps the most extreme is
the use made of general practitioners as a referral source. Nurse therapists
trained at Moorhaven estimate receiving 52 per cent of referrals from
general practitioners whereas for Maudsley-trained nurse therapists this
figure is 22 per cent. Although these data are error prone, i.e. the estimates
are subjective and have not been externally validated, they certainly give
an interesting flavour of the ways nurse therapists believe that work is
organized.

It further seems reasonable to speculate that the particular training centre
at which a nurse therapist is educated is an important determinant of the

Table 11   Estimate of percentage of referrals received from various agencies by
training centre

	Maudsley	Moorhaven	Graylingwell	Total
Psychologists	7.3	2.5	3.5	4.43
GPs	22.0	52.0	28.0	34.0
Social workers	4.5	4.0	2.0	3.5
Nurses	3.0	17.0	15.0	11.66
Psychiatrists	48.0	23.0	33.0	34.66
Others	15.2	1.5	18.5	11.73
Total	100.00	100.00	100.00	99.98

way their work is organized on completion of training. The different emphasis that the three training centres give to the clinical experience of trainees is an area worthy of further research. These data suggest that there is no coherent model for the development of the role of nurse therapists after training, and it seems more likely that each individual nurse therapist adapts to the local service requirements.

The survey revealed that nurse to nurse referrals are not uncommon. On average, it is estimated that nearly 12 per cent of all referrals to nurse therapists come from other nurses. The determination of clinical responsibility for these cases would seem to be a crucial issue. One nurse therapist calculated that some 60 per cent of his referrals came from community psychiatric nurses. Our study did not determine where the clinical responsibility lay in these cases but as nurse to nurse referrals become more common in the future, the issue of clinical responsibility and legal liability should be made less ambiguous.

Patient Contact

The study indicates the essential components of nurse therapist caseload activity after training (see Table 7). Also established are estimates of the time nurse therapists spend in face-to-face clinical work, liaison with other professionals, record-keeping, administration, and research. These results suggest that nurse therapists are able to engage directly in clinical nursing activity for a large proportion of their working week, i.e. 16 hours per week.

The second question, which asked where this clinical activity takes place, is important because it has implications both for the way nurse therapists maintain other professional relationships on completion of training and the advantages and disadvantages implicit in different settings. Table 5 shows that the largest single category of nurse therapists (26 per cent) base their work in community psychiatric nursing departments.

It remains unclear whether nurse therapists are a type of community psychiatric nurse equipped with a specialist clinical skill or wish to regard themselves as a separate professional subgroup. This study indicated that 80.4 per cent of nurse therapists receive no day-to-day clinical supervision, a finding that tends to confirm the impression that nurse therapists do see themselves as a separate subgroup. Although it must be stressed that the concepts of nurse therapist autonomy and independence were originally seen as desirable (Marks et al., 1975).

In an unpublished paper, Lindley et al. (1983) describe the relationship between nurse therapy and clinical supervision. They argue that a lack of formal supervision can enhance the nurse therapist's status as it emphasizes their clinical autonomy. Indeed, an early criticism of the nurse therapy movement was that psychiatric nurses were being trained as mere technicians or psychologists' assistants. However, while this argument was historically a persuasive one, today it begs several questions. During nurse therapy training, clinical supervision of casework is a major teaching element. This survey has demonstrated an abrupt change post-training. The major difficulty is that there is no established mechanism whereby nurse therapists' clinical performance is monitored once alone in the field. While much has been published that demonstrates the efficacy of nurse therapists during training (Marks *et al.*, 1978; Bird *et al.*, 1979) as yet we do not know whether this effectiveness is maintained after qualifying. The lack of formal clinical supervision indicates a level of autonomy certainly but also suggests a degree of professional isolation. Finally, it is possible that the nurse therapists who responded to the question about clinical supervision answered in terms of a need to be seen as autonomous rather than reflecting the actual support that they may receive from colleagues.

In total, this survey's findings begin to build up a composite picture of nurse therapists as independent practitioners, working in a variety of settings, and with few formal supervisory links. The inherent danger in subscribing to this model of practice is that it may become professionally isolating. Nurse therapists seem to be caught in the middle of a no-man's land, between the clinical independence of psychologists and psychiatrists and the mainstream of psychiatric nursing which is currently struggling with the issues of accountability and professionalism. Nurse therapy is now 10 years old and, like community psychiatric nursing in the mid 1960s, at something of a crossroads. Nurse therapists themselves now need to clarify the direction in which they wish to develop. The alternatives are clear, either a closer relationship with psychiatric nursing as a whole, and community psychiatric nurses in particular, or a consolidation of their position as independent practitioners.

What Happens To Nurse Therapists?

On completion of training, nurse therapist trainees are most likely to call themselves 'nurse therapists' and to be paid as charge nurses (see Tables 3 and 4). The pay grades of the remainder, excluding nurse teachers, peak at Nursing Officer. Since most trainees were paid at the charge nurse level during training and, indeed, many were before training, and given that nurse therapists have been in post an average of 3.5 years, the question of whether the acquisition of advanced clinical nursing skills has been at the expense of career advancement must be raised. The question of what level of career advancement is appropriate may be even more pertinent.

There are no easy answers to these questions. It could be argued that, on the one hand, a group of psychiatric nurses have been trained to provide a specialist clinical skill to clients and should not be financially disadvantaged if they wish to continue doing this. On the other hand, the Royal College of Nursing (1981) has stated that nurses who are delivering specialist clinical skills should be paid as sister/charge nurses, although this document suggests considerable flexibility in gradings. A further question is whether it is appropriate for people to remain in clinical practice for a considerable period without any further training. It could be that these issues will be resolved in the next few years by the deliberations of the Pay Review Body.

This survey has shown that nurse therapists feel they have benefited from training, find their current jobs very interesting and see themselves with a similar career in three years time (see page 186). The majority of nurse therapists do not seem likely to undergo any further training. As most of the discussion regarding a clinical career structure in nursing has centred around obtaining further professional qualifications, in almost building-brick fashion, where does this leave the nurse therapist? It is our contention that nurse therapists, through the difficulties of developing corporate identity, have become isolated from current nursing philosophy concerning the direction of professional development. However, this is to some extent understandable given the relatively small numbers of trained nurse therapists and their geographical scatter throughout the country. Unfortunately, there is no one national organization exclusively for nurse therapists. The Royal College of Nursing Behaviour Therapy Forum comes closest to fulfilling this need, but suffers in two ways. Firstly, it is primarily London based which makes attendance for all nurse therapists in the country difficult. Secondly, membership of Forum is extended to all those nurses interested in behaviour therapy and, obviously, attracts others apart from nurse therapists.

Ultimately, what happens in the future to nurse therapists will depend crucially on their ability to organize themselves as a powerful force, in perhaps the same way that community psychiatric nurses have done, through the Community Psychiatric Nurses' Association (CPNA).

Conclusions

This study was originally designed to follow up all trained nurse therapists using simple survey methodology. A questionnaire was constructed which asked straightforward questions about the way nurse therapists were working and how they saw their future. As is usually the case with this kind of survey research, we have ended up asking more questions than we originally posed. However, we feel in a position to offer the following findings:

1   Nurse therapists as a group seem to differ little from other psychiatric nurses taking JBCNS courses in terms of personal and professional characteristics.
2   Nurse therapists organize and locate their work in a wide variety of ways.
3   Nurse therapists overall find their work satisfying and would like to continue working in this kind of clinical specialty, although they feel frustrated at being unable to advance their careers.
4   Nurse therapists state that no-one supervises their day-to-day clinical work, and from their comments seem happy with this state of affairs.

It still remains unclear whether nurse therapists see themselves as pseudo-psychologists, specialist community psychiatric nurses or, indeed, behavioural psychotherapists with no particular professional allegiance. It is our belief that professional involvement is an important issue, because it can lead to an awareness of current professional issues, a means to constant update and revision of clinical practice and the opportunity to influence the direction of one's own specialty.

The survey's findings suggest that nurse therapists' closest professional allies are community psychiatric nurses. The way this relationship develops in the future should be an area of immediate concern for both groups. One obvious possibility is an examination of the way in which the salient elements of both nurse therapist and community psychiatric nurse training programmes could be incorporated.

Finally, nurse therapy has shown itself to be a viable way of treating adult neurotic patients over the past decade. It also seems relevant to question whether this is now the group on which to focus nursing resources. Groups of patients currently being identified as priorities include the elderly mentally ill and the long-stay residents of institutions with chronic problems. In the current economic climate, nurse managers may become reluctant to second nurses to a course that specializes in the treatment of such a small proportion of the total psychiatric population.

To conclude, it is our hope that this preliminary research will act as a springboard to prompt nurse therapists themselves to instigate research that addresses some of the areas we have outlined above, for as Cormack (1983) so aptly summarizes:

Non-practising nurses, researchers and academics are the
principal contributors to the expansion of nursing research and
prescriptive literature in the UK, relatively little data exists
relating to how nurse practitioners view their role and work.

References

Bird, J., Marks, I. M., and Lindley, P. J. (1979). Nurse therapists in psychiatry:
developments, controversies and implications. *British Journal of Psychiatry*,
135, 321–329.
Brooker, C. (1980). The behavioural management of a complex case. *Nursing
Times*, **76**, 367–369.
Brooker, C. and Wiggins, R. D. (1983). Nurse therapist trainee variability: the
implications for selection and training. *Journal of Advanced Nursing*, **8**,
321–328.
Brown, M. (1980). Therapy without pills. *Nursing*, **1**, 810–814.
Cormack, D. (1983). *Psychiatric Nursing Described*. Churchill Livingstone,
Edinburgh.
Daniel, W. W. (1975). Nonresponse in sociological surveys. A review of some
methods for handling the problem. *Sociological Methodology and Research*,
3, 291–307.
Dunkelberg, W. C. and Day, G. S. (1973). Nonresponse bias and call backs in
sample surveys. *Journal of Marketing Research*, **10**, 160–168.
Erdos, P. L. (1970). *Professional Mail Surveys*. McGraw-Hill, New York.
Hall, J. (1979). Nurse therapy and role change in health care professions. *Bulletin
of the British Psychological Society*, **32**, 71–73.
Hoinville, G. and Jowell, R. (1978). *Survey Research Practice*. Heinemann,
London.
Lindley, P. J., Marks, I. M., and McCafferay, F. (1983). National follow up of
nurse therapists. Unpublished.
Marks, I. M., Hallam, R. S., Connolly, J., and Philpott, R. (1977). *Nursing in
Behavioural Psychotherapy*. Royal College of Nursing.
Marks, I. M., Bird, J., and Lindley, P. J. (1978). Psychiatric nurse therapy—
developments and implications. *Behavioural Psychotherapy*, **6**, 25–36.
Millar, E. (1977). Nurse therapy in general practice. *Nursing Mirror*, 12 May,
47–50.
Moser, C. A. and Kalton, G. (1979). *Survey Methods in Social Investigation*.
Heinemann, London.
Nie, N., Hull, C., and Jenkins, J., *et al.* (1970). *Statistical Package for the Social
Sciences*, 2nd edn. McGraw-Hill, New York.
O'Muirchcarraigh, C. and Wiggins, R. D. (1981). The impact of interviewer
variability in an epidemiological survey. *Psychological Medicine*, **2**, 817–824.
Rogers, J. (1983). *The Career Patterns of Nurses who have Completed a J.B.C.N.S.
Certificate*. Joint Board Of Clinical Nursing Studies.
Royal College of Nursing (1981). *A Structure for Nursing*. Royal College of
Nursing.
Sawyer, N. (1983). A fear of cancer. *Nursing Mirror*, **157**, 6–7.

CHAPTER 11

The Behavioural Management of Neurosis by the Psychiatric Nurse Therapist

FRED ROACH and
NANCY FARLEY

Editor's Comments

Fred Roach and Nancy Farley describe in this chapter their careful and systematic study of over 300 patients referred to one nurse behaviour therapist over a three-year period. They utilized pre-treatment, post-treatment, and follow-up measures to monitor and evaluate the effectiveness of the treatment given to patients.

The main value of this study is its clear demonstration of the importance of nurses carefully monitoring their own treatment and outcomes. This study provides a model for practitioners to consider in maintaining careful records of their own work in order to evaluate their effectiveness and monitor the effects of changes in their practice. This is one of the few attempts by psychiatric nurses to record their work systematically.

The researchers are aware of the problems of this type of research design. The absence of a control group means that the possibility of spontaneous recovery unrelated to the treatment cannot be discounted. The lack of other practitioners against whom to compare the results of this one nurse mean that factors specific to this individual may account for the results. It is also impossible to speculate about which aspects of the treatment were beneficial. Factors in the nurse–patient relationship, rather than the behaviour therapy itself, may have brought about the results.

Introduction

As emphasized by Lindley (1980), until the early 1970s the behavioural approach was almost exclusively practised by psychologists and psychiatrists; particularly for those categories of problem where established behavioural methods have been said to be superior to contrasting methods (Marks, 1976). Clinicians who attempt treatment of these problems (obsessive-compulsive disorders, agoraphobia, specific or social phobias, social maladjustment or personality disorders, sexual dysfunction and sexual deviations, as identified by Marks *et al.*, 1978) have often used traditional behavioural therapeutic approaches encompassing a wide range of methods such as desensitization, flooding, exposure, and relaxation. Therapeutic benefit from these approaches is claimed for some 10 per cent of all adult psychiatric out-patients (Marks, 1976) and for about 25 per cent of neurotics (Marks, 1981).

The evidence, however, derives mainly from outcome studies of the behavioural management of neurotics by psychiatrists and psychologists (Eysenck, 1963; Blakemore, 1964; Rachman, 1980; Rachman and Hodgson, 1980; Marks, 1981); scientific evidence of the usefulness of behaviour therapy by the psychiatric nurse therapist is lacking. Behavioural nurse therapists have failed to report their findings. They have allowed others to offer reports (Marks, 1977; Marks *et al.*, 1978), to suggest how psychiatric nurses should function as therapists in the delivery of psychiatric care (Marks *et al.*, 1975; Ginsberg and Marks, 1978) and to present arguments urging the development of a low cost, not so highly educated or trained psychiatric nurse to carry out routine clinical care, so allowing 'highly educated doctors and psychologists to consult on difficult problems, to research and to organize' (Marks, 1981). Such arguments impose limits upon the future growth and development of the psychiatric nurse and ignore the adoption of a nursing model, geared towards a systematic approach to psychiatric nursing care.

This view of the behavioural nurse therapist needs to be challenged. It offers the psychiatric nurse therapist a 'role-as-prescribed' by psychiatrists; a direction guided by the medical model, limiting in function, task-oriented, and an extending role which is characterized by limitations in terms of professional responsibility and autonomy. This therefore, demands further investigation into the usefulness of the psychiatric nurse therapist in the behavioural management of neurosis. The outcome of the behavioural management of neurosis by the psychiatric nurse therapist needs to be reported in terms far more fundamental than 'abundant testimony' (Marks, 1981); 'comments' (Lang, 1977; Chabot, 1979);

'forecast' (Maxmen, 1976); and 'opinion' (Arnold et al., 1977). The aim of this study therefore is to test the hypothesis 'that there is no change in behaviour in neurotics from behaviour therapy by the psychiatric nurse therapist'.

Three hundred and three subjects were referred by consultant psychiatrists, psychologists, social workers, and general practitioners to the psychiatric nurse therapist (second author) between April 1980 and March 1983 for assessment and treatment. Of the 303 subjects (234 (77.22 per cent) females and 69 (22.77 per cent) males) 157 (51.81 per cent) were referred by consultant psychiatrists and 38 (12.54 per cent) were in active therapy other than behavioural. One hundred and eighty-eight (79.99 per cent) were under 45 years of age.

Method

A simple design without control groups was considered sufficient for this study. Once referred, subjects were offered an appointment to be seen by the psychiatric nurse therapist (who is specially trained in the use of behavioural techniques) either at the nurse therapist's surgery or in their own home, dependent upon 'problem-referred'. Sixteen (5.28 per cent) refused treatment, 34 (11.22 per cent) failed to keep the appointment, and 18 (5.94 per cent) were unsuitable for behaviour therapy. These 68 (22.45 per cent) were referred back to the appropriate referring agent. Two hundred and thirty-five (77.56 per cent) agreed to behavioural treatment and were accepted by the psychiatric nurse therapist. Table 1 shows the sex distribution and response category of the 303 subjects referred.

Subjects

Two hundred and thirty-five subjects, 174 (74.05 per cent) females and 61 (25.95 per cent) males completed behavioural treatment by the

Table 1   Sex distribution and response category of 303 subjects referred

Response category	Male	Female	Total	Percentage
Refused treatment	3	13	16	5.28
Failed to keep appointment	4	30	34	11.22
Unsuitable for behavioural therapy	1	17	18	5.94
Agreed to behavioural treatment	61	174	235	77.56
	69	234	303	100%

psychiatric nurse therapist. Forty-three (18.29 per cent) were under 25 years of age, 145 (61.70 per cent) were between 25 and 44 years of age and 47 (20 per cent) were 45 years of age or above. Table 2 shows the age and sex distribution of the subjects.

All subjects that were referred had been diagnosed as manifesting problems characteristic of neuroses for which treatment by behaviour therapy would seem suitable. Subjects were then systematically assessed by the nurse therapist as a way of identifying problems, setting targets, implementing and evaluating therapy, in the application of behavioural principles.

Table 2   Age and sex distribution of 235 subjects who completed behavioural treatment by the psychiatric nurse therapist

Age	Male	Female	Total	Percentage
Under 25 years	7	36	43	18.30
25–44 years	42	103	145	61.70
45 and above	12	35	47	20
	61	174	235	100%

Table 3   Sex distribution of subjects: problems suitable for behaviour therapy by the psychiatric nurse therapist

Identified problem referred	Males	Females	Total	Percentage
Agoraphobia	9	48	57	24.25
Social anxiety	15	13	28	11.91
Specific phobia	2	10	12	5.10
Obsessions	6	16	22	9.36
Body pain/headaches	1	4	5	2.12
Marital	2	7	9	3.82
Sexual	1	6	7	2.97
Social maladjustment	23	63	86	36.59
Habit disorder	0	2	2	00.85
Stammer	1	1	2	00.85
Claustrophobia	1	1	2	00.85
Dietary	0	3	3	1.27
	61	174	235	99.94

Procedure

Behavioural analysis (Kanfer and Saslow, 1969) of subjects' problem-referred identified twelve problems to be treated. Table 3 shows the sex distribution of subjects in terms of problems identified as suitable for behavioural management. Of the problems identified for behavioural treatment, social maladjustment affected the largest number of subjects, 86 (36.59 per cent). Agoraphobia affected 57 (24.25 per cent) and social anxiety 28 (11.91 per cent). Obsessions affected 22 (9.36 per cent).

For treatment purposes, subjects' problem-referred was placed in one of five groups of 'problems identified to be treated behaviourally'. These five groups were: phobias, anxiety, marital and sexual, obsessions, and social maladjustment. Table 4 shows the distribution of 'problem-referred' to 'problem treated'. The preference was for observable, measurable aspects of behaviour with concern for the nature of the problem, its duration and its intensity.

Prior to the start of behavioural management, subjects completed a Life History Questionnaire which drew more attention to the nature of their problem and pointed to their expectations from therapy. A behavioural interview was then carried out with the subject. The aim of this was to detect the subject's conceptualization of the problem and to assist with

Table 4   Distribution of groups from problem referred to problem treated

Problem referred groups	Males	Females	Total	Percentage	Problem treated groups
Agoraphobia	9	48	57	24.25	
Specific phobia	2	10	12	5.10	
Claustrophobia	1	1	2	0.85	
	12	59	71	30.2	Phobia
Social anxiety	15	13	28	11.91	
Body pain	1	4	5	2.12	
Habit disorder	0	2	2	0.85	
Stammer	1	1	2	0.85	
Dietary	0	3	3	1.27	
	17	23	40	17.0	Anxiety
Marital	2	7	9	3.82	
Sexual	1	6	7	2.97	
	3	13	16	6.8	Marital and Sexual
Obsessions	6	16	22	9.36	Obsessions
Social maladjustment	23	63	86	36.5	Social maladjustment

its formulation by psychiatric nurse therapist. Next, baseline measurements were established through various measures (Rearley *et al.*, 1978) in the form of self-rating questionnaires. These were recorded to aid the planning, implementation, and evaluation of therapy with the subject. Behavioural targets were then set and individual treatment plans agreed between

Table 5   Treatment procedure

Problem treated	Behavioural management	Reference
Agoraphobia	Exposure *in vivo* and anxiety management	Emmelkamp *et al.*, 1978
Claustrophobia	Exposure *in vivo* and cognitive therapy	Suinn and Richardson, 1971
Specific phobia	Participant modelling	Bandura, *et al.*, 1974
Social anxiety	Assertive and social skills training	Alberi and Emmon, 1973 Trower, *et al.*, 1978
Body pain	Relaxation	Jacobson, 1938
Habit disorder	Habit reversal	Azrin and Nunn, 1973
Stammering	Habit reversal	Azrin and Nunn, 1974
Dietary	Cognitive behavioural approach to bulimia nervosa	Fairburn, 1981
Marital	Conjoint marital therapy	Crowe, 1973
Sexual	Sex therapy. Counselling for sexual problem	Masters and Johnson, 1970 Greenwood and Bancroft, 1977
Obsessions	Satiation. Thought stopping exposure and response prevention	Stern, 1978
Social maladjustment	Non-specific behaviour therapy for anxiety control	Suinn and Richardson, 1971
Social	Relaxation	Jacobson, 1938
Maladjustment	Cognitive restructing	Goldfried *et al.*, 1974
Maladjustment	Stress innovation	Meichenbaum, 1973
Maladjustment	Self-instruction	Meichenbaum, 1973

Table 6   Number of therapy sessions* and hours for problem treated

Problem treated	n	Sessions	Mean	Hours	Mean
Phobia	71	725	10.21	543.75	7.65
Anxiety	40	384	9.6	288	7.2
Marital and sexual	16	119	7.43	89.25	5.57
Obsessions	22	226	10.27	169.5	7.70
Social maladjustment	86	440	5.22	330.00	3.83

*Therapy sessions lasted from 45 minutes to two hours.

the therapist and the subject. Treatment then followed as outlined in Table 5. The average therapy time for each of the five problems treated was recorded (see table 6).

Uniform and Specific Measures of Problem Treated

Uniform measurement of target problems was carried out on 0–8 scales where 0 scored no problem and 8 scored maximum disability. This was done at the start of treatment, at the end of treatment, and at three months follow-up for each of the five problems treated. Decrease in problem severity, as measured, established new goals which, when achieved, decreased behavioural management (Rearley and Gilbert, 1976) and led to the subject's discharge and follow-up programme. Outcome was recorded in terms of failure, improvement or success. As specific measures the phobia anxiety and avoidance scales (Watson and Marks, 1971) were used, in addition, for testing change of behaviour in the specific problems — phobias, anxiety, and obsessions — so that correlations could be made with the results from uniform measures.

Apparatus

A tape recorder was used to record interviews with subjects and to introduce certain behavioural management strategies. Selected video tapes were used with some subjects (phobias). Stop watches were used to monitor some subject's progress in certain behavioural situations.

Results

Follow-up data were compared with those at pre-behavioural management and post-behavioural management, using two-tailed t-test (related). Improvement since pre-behavioural management by the psychiatric nurse therapist was significant on the phobia anxiety scales and the phobia avoidance scales for social anxiety and phobias. (The results for agoraphobia as a separate group ($n = 57$) was not significant on the phobia anxiety scales — other phobia ($t = 0.88$, df 56, $p > 0.05$).) For obsessions, improvement was significant on phobia avoidance scales — main phobia ($t = 3.01$, df 21 $p < 0.05$) (see Table 7).

The improvement manifested between post-behavioural management and follow-up at three months was significant on the phobia anxiety scales and phobia avoidance scales for the phobias. Agoraphobia as a separate group showed significance on phobia anxiety scales — main phobias and

Table 7 Effects of behavioural management by the psychiatric nurse therapist at three months follow-up

Problem treated	Variables	Pre-behavioural management		Follow-up		df	t	p
		Mean	S.D.	Mean	S.D.			
Obsessions	Phobia anxiety:							
	main phobia	6.59	3.47	2.45	2.97	21	5.31	<0.001
	other phobia	6.63	2.56	2.25	1.60	21	5.55	<0.001
	Phobia avoidance:							
	main phobia	5.90	4.70	1.69	1.07	21	3.01	<0.05
	other phobia	7.36	2.65	1.72	2.69	21	11.54	<0.001
Social anxiety	Phobia anxiety:							
	main phobia	8.00	3.72	1.71	2.14	27	4.05	<0.001
	other phobia	5.48	4.59	1.90	1.05	27	7.09	<0.001
	Phobia avoidance:							
	main phobia	6.00	1.85	1.70	1.39	27	6.25	<0.001
	other phobia	6.60	2.08	0.78	1.04	27	8.86	<0.001
Phobias	Phobia anxiety:							
	main phobia	6.63	2.17	2.37	1.11	70	4.03	<0.001
	other phobia	6.06	1.90	2.26	1.08	70	14.35	<0.001
	Phobia avoidance:							
	main phobia	6.98	2.62	2.50	1.18	70	9.61	<0.001
	other phobia	6.88	1.74	2.56	0.21	70	12.80	<0.001

Table 8 Effects of behavioural management by the psychiatric nurse therapist following completion of treatment at 3 months follow-up

Problem treated	Variables	Post-behavioural management		Follow-up				
		Mean	S.D.	Mean	S.D.	df	t	p
Obsessions	Phobia anxiety:							
	main phobia	3.45	1.82	2.45	2.97	21	1.47	N.S.
	other phobia	3.16	3.53	2.25	1.60	21	2.44	<0.05
	Phobia avoidance:							
	main phobia	3.57	3.23	1.69	1.07	21	2.44	<0.05
	other phobia	3.00	2.50	1.72	2.69	21	2.62	<0.05
Social anxiety	Phobia anxiety:							
	main phobia	3.26	3.74	1.71	2.14	27	2.61	<0.05
	other phobia	3.13	4.59	1.90	1.05	27	2.95	<0.05
	Phobia avoidance:							
	main phobia	3.26	2.15	1.70	1.39	27	3.83	<0.001
	other phobia	2.21	1.43	0.78	1.04	27	3.50	<0.05
Phobias	Phobia anxiety:							
	main phobia	3.11	2.90	2.37	1.11	70	4.51	<0.001
	other phobia	3.73	3.08	2.26	1.08	70	4.54	<0.001
	Phobia avoidance:							
	main phobia	4.01	3.12	2.50	1.18	70	3.75	<0.001
	other phobia	2.70	2.54	2.56	0.21	70	3.70	<0.001

other phobias ($t = 2.92$, df 56 $p < 0.01$ and $t = 2.93$, df 56 $p < 0.01$, respectively) and on phobias avoidance scales — main phobia and other phobias ($t = 2.91$, df 56 $p < 0.01$ and $t = 2.29$, df 56 $p < 0.05$, respectively). For anxiety, there was significance on phobia avoidance scales — main phobias ($t = 3.83$, df 27 $p < 0.001$) but for obsessions, the level of significance varied on the various scales (see Table 8).

Chi-square

Chi-square tests for significance of outcome, in terms of failure, improvement or success of behavioural management, between the results from the behavioural management subjects' self-rating target measure, the nurse therapist's global rating of psychiatric state, and the improvement at follow-up on the phobia anxiety and avoidance scales (for obsessions, anxiety, social maladjustment) were calculated. Improvement from behavioural management by the psychiatric nurse therapist was found to be significant in all the problems treated apart from phobias ($\chi^2 = 6.56$, df2 $p < 0.05$) (see Table 9).

Table 9   Effects of behavioural management by the psychiatric nurse therapist in terms of outcome

Problem treated	No improve- ment	Some improve- ment	Complete improve- ment	df	χ^2	p
Phobias	25	13	33	2	6.564	n.s.
Anxiety	9	15	16	2	2.149	<0.05
Marital and sexual	9	2	5	2	2.589	<0.05
Obsessions	12	3	7	2	5.546	<0.05
Social maladjustment	29	28	29	2	0.023	<0.05

A further test for significance of the outcome of behaviour therapy by the nurse on 235 subjects was calculated, using grouped data. The results were found to be significant ($\chi^2 = 14.503$, df8, $p < 0.05$), which in general terms indicated that the psychiatric nurse therapist's use of behavioural techniques in the management of some neurotic problems had been effective.

Uniform and Specific Measurement Results

The results of uniform measurement by the psychiatric nurse of target problem as shown on 0–8 scales, as related to the phobic anxiety and

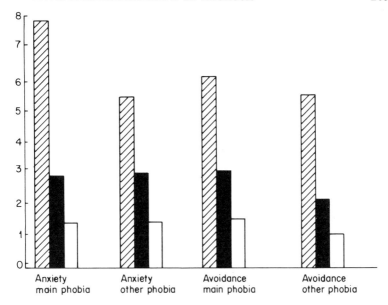

Figure 1   Obsessions: mean scores on phobia anxiety and avoidance scales (pre-behavioural management, post-behavioural management, follow-up)

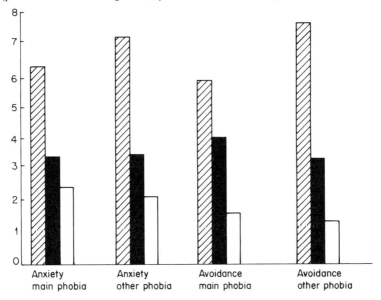

Figure 2   Anxiety: mean scores on phobia anxiety and avoidance scales (pre-behavioural management, post-behavioural management, follow-up)

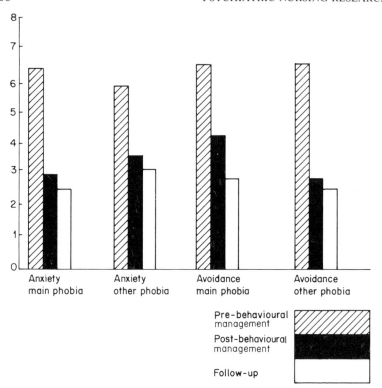

Figure 3   Phobias: mean scores on phobia anxiety and avoidance scales (pre-behavioural management, post behavioural management, follow-up)

avoidance scales at pre-behavioural management, post-behavioural management, and follow-up by the psychiatric nurse, are shown in Figure 1, 2, and 3 for obsessions, anxiety, and phobias, respectively.

Over half, 58.57 per cent, of subjects tested on phobia anxiety and avoidance scales were found to have improved on the main phobia at follow-up, thus showing a reduction of the main phobia by about one point on the 0–8 scale. A similar pattern of change in behaviour was shown for both the marital and sexual and social maladjustment groups using other measures.

Discussion

The results of this study show that the improvements shown in behaviour by neurotics following behavioural management by the nurse therapist were, after three months, being maintained; 38.29 per cent of the subjects had completely recovered and 25.95 per cent were responding favourably to the behavioural management of their problem.

These results suggest that some 64.24 per cent of neurotics benefited from behavioural treatments of their problem by the psychiatric nurse. Earlier reports (Marks, 1976; Marks, 1981) claimed that 10–25 per cent of neurotics benefited from such treatments. It must be borne in mind, however, that these studies were more concerned with the behavioural management of neurotics by psychiatrists and psychologists and therefore cannot be easily compared with outcome studies by nurse therapists. Likewise the finding of psychiatrists and psychologists cannot be readily compared with the findings of this study.

The treatment of phobias is directly relevant to this point. Some reports suggest that behaviour therapy is the treatment of choice for phobic disorders (Marks, 1981; Wilson, 1981). The technique used, in most cases, is 'exposure' which is seen as capable of reducing fear (Bandura et al., 1974; Kazdin and Wilson, 1978; Marks, 1975; Marks, 1978; Rachman and Wilson, 1980; Wolpe, 1958; Wolpe, 1973). Bandura et al.'s (1977) persuasive theory, however, denies the claim that exposure is a necessary condition for fear reduction and suggests that the more dependable the source of information the greater the changes in self-efficacy. DeSilva and Rachman (1981) also argue that dependable sources of information of whatever form can lead to fear reduction. The results of tests of significance on a group of phobic patients in this study showed no significant change in patients' behaviour from behaviour therapy in which exposure was involved. Marks (1981) acknowledges that exposure treatments may ultimately be working by teaching patients coping skills which can be acquired without direct professional intervention. There is growing awareness also that the management of phobias need not involve the trained professional. Psychiatric nurse therapists therefore need to be more aware that many phobias can be helped by self-help groups, manuals or by the patient working alone. This implies that the nurse therapist should be more mindful of the amount of time spent helping this type of patient with their problem. In this study the average time spent with the phobias ($n = 71$) was 7.65 hours for each individual person, and of this group 57 (47 female, 10 male) perceived agoraphobia as their problem. The females constituted 82.45 per cent of this group, thus comparing favourably with the view that 75 per cent of agoraphobics are female (Agras et al., 1969; Marks, 1969).

More recently attention has been paid to the lack of agreement on a definition of the term 'anxiety' (Daly, 1978) as used to describe an emotional state (Spielberger, 1969). It is not worthwhile exploring such controversies here but the behavioural management of the anxiety problem in general proved most successful for the nurse therapists and would seem to suggest that it is in this area that nurse therapists should devote more time. However, when 'social anxiety' as a separate group was considered it appeared that, like agoraphobias, it is a behaviour which could be managed in the absence of the therapist. How then can it be justifiable to train therapists to manage behaviourally conditions which in reality do not require such interventions? Psychiatric nurse therapists, it would seem, ought to concentrate their efforts more on those whose problems fall within such areas as body pain, habit disorder, stuttering, dietary disorders, marital and sexual problems, and anxiety. The behavioural nurse therapist was most successful helping patients to overcome these problems. Perhaps the use of positive self-talk (Bandura et al., 1969) is an important factor in achieving positive outcomes. It would therefore seem more useful to train behaviour nurse therapists in the use of such skills.

Marks (1975) showed that obsessional patients whose behaviour changed in the desired direction, but whose attitudes remained unaltered had, at follow-up, reverted to their pre-therapy behaviours. It may be assumed that in the early stages of therapy the behaviour of those obsessionals who failed (39.81 per cent) changed, but attitudes may not have altered (Hersen, 1973).

Overall, the results from data analysis show that the behavioural management of neurosis by the psychiatric nurse is effective only in certain conditions in particular social maladjustment, and less effective in others such as phobias and social anxiety. Sloane et al. (1975) found behavioural treatments significantly more effective with clients who presented with severe neurotic problems. It would seem from the findings of this study that phobic and social anxiety problems are not so severe and that these patients ought to be referred to self-help groups or self-help manuals. Claims to the effectiveness of these has already been noted (Kass and Stauss, 1975). In short, it seems that these problems can be managed without direct professional intervention (Marks, 1980). However, as Wilson (1981) suggested the evidence so far remains insufficient. Behavioural nurse therapists need to engage in more purposeful research which would provide more direct answers to many of the questions raised in this study.

In summary, it is difficult to assess the effectiveness of any therapy (Rearley and Gilbert, 1979) or indeed any therapist, given the interplay of external variables which may be difficult to control. It is equally difficult to make claims to the effectiveness of behaviour therapy with neurotics by the psychiatric nurse therapist because variables other than those related to behavioural intervention by the nurse may be acting upon the problem the patient brings to the situation, to produce the subsequent behavioural changes which come to be labelled success. There is also the possibility that what is generally described as 'behaviour therapy' by psychiatrists or psychologists is different from that practised by the psychiatric nurse. This view rests upon the belief that a retention of the principles upon which behaviourism is formulated and adherence to a procedural format does not necessarily give authority to claims that behaviour therapy as managed by the psychiatrist or by the psychologist is the same when managed by the psychiatric nurse therapist who might in reality be doing something else.

References

Agras, W. A., Aylvester, D., and Oliveau, D. (1969). The epidemiology of common fears and phobias. *Comprehensive Psychiat.*, **10**, 151–156.
Alberi, R. E. and Emmon, M. (1973). *Your Perfect Right.*
Arnold, E., Barnaby, N., McManus, J., and Smeltzer, D. J. (1977). Prevention by specific perceptual remediation for vulnerable first graders. *Archives of General Psychiatry*, **34**, 1279–1294.
Azrin, N. H. and Nunn, R. G. (1973). Habit reversal: A method of eliminating nervous habits and tics. *Behavioural Research and Therapy*, **11**, 619–628.
Azrin, N. H. and Nunn, R. G. (1974). A rapid method of eliminating stuttering by a regulated breathing approach. *Behavioural Research and Therapy*, **12**, 279–286.
Bandura, A., Blanchard, E. B., and Ritter, B. (1969). The relative efficacy of desensitization and modelling approaches for including behavioural, affective, and attitudinal changes. *J. Person. Soc. Psychol.*, **13**, 173–199.
Bandura, A., Jeffery, R. W., and Wright, C. L. (1974). Efficiency of participant modelling as a function of response induction aids. *J. Abnormal Psycho.*, **83**, 56–64.
Blakemore, C. B. (1964). The application of behaviour therapy to a sexual disorder, in H. J. Eysenck (Ed.), *Experiments in Behaviour Therapy*. Pergamon, Oxford.
Chabot, B. (1979) The right to care for each other and its silent erosion. *Tidschrift voor Psychotherapie*, **5**, 199–216.
Crowe, M. J. (1973). Conjoint marital therapy: advice or interpretation? *Journal of Psychosomatic Research*, **17**, 309–315.
Daly, S. (1978). Behavioural correlates of social anxiety. *British Journal of Social and Clinical Psychology*, **17**, 117–120.
DeSilva, P. and Rachman, S. (1981). Is exposure a necessary condition for fear-reduction? *Behavioural Research and Therapy*, **19**, 227–232.
Emmelkamp, P., Kuipers, A., and Eggeraat, J. (1978). Cognitive modification vs prolonged exposure *in vivo*: a comparison with agoraphobics. *Behavioural Research and Therapy*, **16**, 33–41.
Eysenck, H. J. (1963). Behaviour therapy, extinction and relapse in neurosis. *British Journal Psychiat.*, **109**, 112–118.

Fairburn, C. (1981). A Cognitive behavioural approach to the management of bulimia. *Psychological Medicine*, **11**, 707–711.

Ginsberg, G. and Marks, I. M. (1978). Costs and benefits of behavioural psychotherapy. A pilot study of neurotics treated by nurse-therapists. *Psychological Medicine*.

Goldfried, M., Decenteceo, E., and Weinberg, L. (1974). Systematic rational restructing as a self control technique. *Behaviour Therapy*, **5**, 247–254.

Greenwood, J. and Bancroft, J. (1977). *Counselling for Sexual Problems*.

Hersen, M. (1973). Developments in behaviour modification. *Journal of Nervous and Mental Diseases*, **156**, 373–376.

Jacobson, E. (1938). *Progressive Relaxation*. University of Chicago Press, Chicago.

Kanfer, F. H. and Saslow, G. (1969). Behavioural diagnosis, in C. M. Franks (Ed.), *Behaviour Therapy: Appraisal and Status*, McGraw-Hill, New York.

Kass, D. J. and Stauss, F. F. (1975). *Sex Therapy at Home*. Simon and Schuster, New York.

Kazdin, A. E. and Wilson, G. T. (1978). *Evaluation of Behaviour Therapy: Issues, Evidence, and Research Strategies*. Ballinger, Cambridge, Massachusetts.

Lang, P. J. (1977). Imagery in therapy. *Behaviour Therapy*.

Lindley, P. (1980). Behavioural approaches. *Medical Education*, pp. 808–809.

Marks, I. M. (1969). *Fears and Phobias*. Heinemann Medical Books, London.

Marks, I. M. (1975). Behaviour treatments of phobic and obsessive-compulsive disorders: A Critical appraisal, in M. Hersen, R. M. Eisler, and P. M. Miller (Eds), *Progress in Behaviour Modification*, vol. 1, Academic Press, New York.

Marks, I. M. (1976). The current status of behavioural psychotherapy: Theory and practice. *American Journal Psychiat.*, **133**, 253.

Marks, I. M. (1977). Exposure treatments, in S. Agras (Ed.), *Behaviour Modification*, 2nd edn. Little Brown and Co, New York.

Marks, I. M. (1978). Behavioural psychotherapy of adult neurosis, in S. Garfield and A. E. Bergin (Eds) Handbook of Psychotherapy and Behaviour Modification, 2nd edn. Wiley, Chichester.

Marks, I. M. (1980). *Living with Fear*. McGraw-Hill, New York.

Marks, I. M. (1981). Behavioural concepts and treatments of neuroses. *Behavioural Psychotherapy*, **9**, 137–154.

Marks, I. M., Bird, J., and Lindley, P. (1978) Behavioural nurse therapists 1978 — developments and implications. *Behavioural Psychotherapy*, **6**, 25–36.

Marks, I. M., Connolly, J. C., Hallam, R. S., and Philpott, R. (1975). Nurse therapists in behavioural psychotherapy. *British Medical Journal*, **3**, 144–148.

Masters, W. H. and Johnson, V. (1970). *Human Sexual Inadequacy*. Churchill, London.

Maxmen, J. S. (1976). *The Post-physician Era: Medicine in the 21st Century*. Wiley, New York.

Meichenbaum, D. (1973). A Self instructural approach to stress management: A proposal for stress inoculation training, in C. Spielberger and I. Sanason (Eds), *Stress and Anxiety*, vol. 2, Wiley, New York.

Rachman, S. (1980) Emotional processing. *Behavioural Research and Therapy*, **18**, 51–60.

Rachman, S. and Hodgson, R. J. (1980). *Obsessions and Compulsions*. Prentice-Hall, Englewood Cliffs, New Jersey.

Rachman, S. and Wilson, G. T. (1980). *The Effects of Psychological Therapy*. Pergamon, Oxford.

Rearley, W. and Gilbert, M. T. (1976). The behavioural treatment approach to potential child abuse — two illustrative cases. *Social Work Today*, **76**, 166–168.

Rearley, W., Gilbert, M. T., and Carver, V. (1978). The behavioural approach to child abuse (2), in V. Carver (Ed.), *Child Abuse: A Study Text*. Open University Press, Milton Keynes.

Rearley, W. and Gilbert, M. T. (1979). The analysis and treatment of child abuse by behavioural psychotherapy. *Child Abuse and Neglect*, vol. 3, Pergamon Press, Oxford, pp. 509–514.

Spielberger, C. D. (1969). Theory and research on anxiety, in C. D. Spielberger (Ed.), *Anxiety and Behaviour*. Academic Press, New York.

Sloane, R. B., Staples, F. R., Cristol, A. H., Yorkston, N. J., and Whipple, K. (1975). *Psychotherapy Versus Behaviour Therapy*. Harvard University Press, Cambridge, Massachusetts.

Stern, R. S. (1978). Obsessive thoughts: the problem of therapy. *British Journal Psychiat.*, **132**, 200–205.

Suinn, R. M., and Richardson, F. (1971). Anxiety management training: A non-specific behaviour therapy programme for anxiety control. *Behaviour Therapy*, **2**, 498–510.

Watson, J. P. and Marks, I. M. (1971). Relevant and irrelevant fear in flooding: a cross-over study of phobic patients. *Behavioural Therapy*, **2**, 275–293.

Wilson, G. T. (1981). Behavioural Concepts and Treatment of Neurosis: Comments on Marks. *Behavioural Psychotherapy*, **9**, 155–166.

Wolpe, J. (1958). *Psychotherapy by Reciprocal Inhibition*. Stanford University Press, Stanford, California.

Wolpe, J. (1973). *The Practice of Behaviour Therapy*, 2nd edn. Pergamon Press, New York.

Part E   Community Psychiatric Nursing

CHAPTER 12

Factors Influencing General Practitioners to Refer Patients to Community Psychiatric Nurses

EDWARD WHITE

Editor's Comments

In this interesting and complex study, Edward White used multiple research techniques to examine various aspects of the relationship between general practitioners (GPs) and community psychiatric nurses (CPNs). He found a great diversity among GPs in attitudes towards psychologically distressed patients, management strategies, and practices in relation to referral of patients to CPNs. Relationships with and referrals to CPNs seemed to be at least partly a function of the relationships negotiated between the individuals concerned. This chapter also includes a valuable account of the historical development of the CPN service.

Introduction

Developments in General Practice

The term general practitioner (GP) came into use in the United Kingdom at about the beginning of the nineteenth century. Medical practice before that time had been sharply divided into three categories: physicians, surgeons, and apothecaries in a system which had remained stable for 200 years. The professional and social gulf between each group was carefully circumscribed. The GP evolved from all three branches of the medical profession which, of itself has created a problem for general practice which has lasted for more than a hundred years (Drury and Hull, 1979). Friction between the competing groups of doctors has characterized the historical development of the GP and the latter part of the nineteenth and twentieth centuries have been occupied by the careful construction of divisions between those doctors who worked in hospitals and did specialist work and those who did not work in hospitals and remained generalists. Bowling (1981) has argued that GPs became part of a unified medical profession at the expense of remaining at the bottom of the medical hierarchy; their status currently as uncertain as their role. Further, that despite many official and government reports which attempted to provide it, the problem of general practice still seemed to be its lack of role definition based on an independent body of knowledge — a prerequisite of full professional status. By the late 1950s, dissatisfaction among GPs had assumed considerable proportions which, Brearley et al. (1978) argued, had not been removed by the founding of the College of General Practitioners in 1953. Although measures which followed the Report of the Royal Commission on Doctors' and Dentists' Remuneration (Pilkington, 1960) increased the earnings of GPs and modestly stimulated the development of larger group practices, the image of general practice was not improved by the changes and little had been done to bridge the gap between primary and specialist services. The recent and substantial increase in the proportion of GPs who have attended courses or continuing education has not altered the feeling of isolation among them (Cartwright and Anderson, 1981). Moreover, the post-war changes in the pattern of health care provision ran counter to the assumption that the burden of management of one aspect of general practice, psychiatric work, would shift from primary care to specialist services; from general practitioner to psychiatrist.

The single most significant shift of emphasis in the provision of psychiatric care from the institution to the community was provided in 1961 by the then Minister of Health. His announcement (Powell, 1961) that the Conservative Government intended to reduce by half, and by 1975, the 150 000 mental hospital beds in the National Health Service (NHS) prompted Titmuss (1961) to argue immediately that the new policy, which has since been reflected in government enquiries connected with the health service (DHSS 1975, 1976, 1981a), was based on rather limited statistics of doubtful interpretation. Moreover, it implied a quite remarkable degree of optimism in the capacity and willingness of GPs to participate in community care.

The recent encouragement for GPs to secure more training in the psychological aspects of medicine (Merrison, 1979; Royal College of General Practitioners, 1981) acknowledged an unwillingness and unpreparedness of some GPs to deal with that aspect of general practice

(Rawnsley and Lounden, 1962; Walton, 1966; May and Gregory, 1968; Reynolds and Bice, 1971; Johnson, 1973, 1974; Clyne, 1974). More recently Cartwright and Anderson (1981) found GPs to be increasingly busy and that this was associated with their perception of a relatively high proportion of the consultations as being trivial, inappropriate or unnecessary. One source of this feeling seemed to be the seeking of advice by patients about family, social, and psychological problems.

By the end of the 1960s, it had become clear, nevertheless, that the GP was coping with an overwhelming proportion of the total amount of psychiatric morbidity in the community. The primacy of the GP in the context of practice can be seen by the fact that 98 per cent of the population are registered with an NHS GP, of whom 60–70 per cent consult at least once in any one year (Williams, 1979). Further, about one person in four of the population experiences some form of psychological disturbance during the course of one year, as detected by the General Health Questionnaire (Goldberg and Blackwell, 1970) although it might be transient, non-specific, and self-limiting. Fractionally less than one person in four (23 per cent) of the population will present at a GP's surgery with some form of psychological disturbance on at least one occasion during one year, although this too may be transient, non-specific, and self-limiting. A little over one person in seven (14 per cent) of attenders who so present at the doctor's surgery, will have a measure of perceptable disturbance detected at least once during one year by GPs. About one in twenty of all illnesses are referred to a psychiatrist (Goldberg and Huxley, 1980; Goldberg, 1982). GPs therefore manage about 95 per cent of conspicuous psychiatric morbidity without recourse to psychiatrist referral. Thus as Williams (1979) suggested, two distinct GP–psychiatrist interfaces could be recognized. Firstly, that which centred around referral and the transfer of clinical responsibility from GP to psychiatrist and, secondly, that which concerned the way in which GP and psychiatrist could work together to provide optimum psychiatric care for patients who were not referred to psychiatrists and who remained primarily the responsibility of the general practitioner. However, a recent national development in the United Kingdom has offered a contribution to the management of psychologically distressed patients beyond the conventional dichotomy; direct GP referral to a community psychiatric nurse (CPN).

Developments in Community Psychiatric Nursing

In July 1954, two qualified mental nurses were seconded to extramural duties in the London Borough of Croydon whose population of 250 000 was served by Warlingham Park Hospital, Surrey, England. The out-patient nurses, as they were later to be known, kept contact between the hospital and discharged patients to help 're-establish' them in the community. The scheme began because of a shortage of psychiatric social workers to relieve the pressure on beds and 'thus reduce overcrowding with a consequent better service to patients within the hospital' (Moore, 1961; May and Moore, 1963; May, 1965). Three years later at Moorhaven Hospital, Devon, a similar service 'just started' from a recognition by social workers and medical staff that a nurse was 'the person best fitted to care for certain patients in the community' (Hunter, 1959; Greene, 1968).

What began as an experiment in 1954 has since developed into a national network of some 219 separate CPN services, 92 per cent of them having been established since 1970 (Community Psychiatric Nurses Association, 1981). From 1974, the then Joint Board of Clinical Nursing Studies (now the English National Board of the United Kingdom Central Council for Nursing, Midwifery and Health Visiting) has been responsible for the Post-Registered Mental Nurse training of CPNs and has validated eight centres to provide the academic year long, non-mandatory, course in the principles and practice of community psychiatric nursing, psychology, sociology, and social administration.

The prevailing educational model has lent itself to the development of a CPN role popularly characterized by Barker (1981). Within his paradigm, the role is argued to contain four elements: assessor and therapist to patients and relatives, consultant to other professionals, and clinician to monitor the wide range of psychotropic drugs. Jones *et al.* (1978) has suggested that the 1960s community care policy relied chiefly on the effect of the then new range of psychotropic drugs introduced in the mid 1950s. The administration of such preparations has long been regarded the *sine qua non* of community psychiatric nursing and has provided an indicator of the predominant client group, operational base, and referral source with which CPNs have been historically linked; respectively, previously hospitalized individuals with disorders alleviated by the regular injection of those substances, particularly those with schizophrenia as a diagnosis (Warren 1971, Hunter 1978), the psychiatric hospital, and the psychiatrist.

More recently, the trend has moved markedly toward a closer identifi-cation with primary care givers (Shaw 1975, Harker *et al.*, 1976; Corser and Ryer, 1977; Sencicle, 1981). By 1981, it was reported that only 27 per cent of CPN services had retained a psychiatrist-only referral system and more than half had their main bases outside psychiatric hospitals (Community Psychiatric Nurses Association, 1981). Griffith and Mangen (1980) reported that the overall view which emerged from their review was that the psychiatric hospital was gradually becoming only one source of treatment rather than the sole locus of it. However, Brook and Cooper (1975) argued that there was no simple formula for strengthening the primary health care team in its management of mental health disorders. This was dependent on the type of community, the resources available, and on the training and attitudes of the different professional workers.

Psychiatric referral

The role of the GP, therefore, in the assessment and treatment of this aspect of treatment has remained important, particularly since the Second World War, occupying the intermediate position between the community and specialist services. However, as Robertson (1979) reported, in psychiatry, probably more than any other branch of medicine, there was greater variation in the types of patients GPs were able and prepared to treat themselves and those whom they referred. The clinical condition of the patient might be thought of as being of prime importance in determining whether referral was made, but there was considerable evidence to suggest this was not so (Kessel, 1960; Walton, 1969; Kaeser and Cooper, 1971). Further, while it has been known that some demographic characteristics of the patient, such as age, sex, and marital status affect the chances of referral (Shepherd *et al.*, 1966) they could not solely account for the variation in referral rates by different GPs. As Goldberg and Huxley (1980) have put it, the differences between them reside not in their patients but in the GP's different concepts of psychiatric disorder and the threshold they adopt for case identification. While little was known about what determined a GP's decision to refer a patient to a psychiatrist, still less was known—from the inchoate nature of the research—of the influences on decisions to refer to a community psychiatric nurse.

The Specifics of the Study

An exploratory study, part of which is presently described, therefore attempted to contribute more information about the developing relationship on the basis of an examination of the work demands made by all 68 GPs upon six community psychiatric nurses working within one Health District in the South East of England. The resident population was 148 000. About three-quarters of the population lived in an urban environment, while the remainder lived in almost entirely rural settings.

The 68 GPs qualified as doctors between 1941 and 1977, the average then being a little over 21 years ago. Fifty-two practised in the urban areas. Thirteen were single practitioners, twelve worked in pairs while twenty-four worked in eight groups of three. There were two groups of four and one group each of five and six. Fifty-eight (85 per cent) of the GPs were male.

Each of the six CPN's were identified with particular GP practices and worked with, on average, eleven general practitioners located in three to four practices. Of the six CPNs, one had been specifically trained as a community psychiatric nurse. This accorded closely with the national picture of 15 per cent found by Dunnell and Dobbs (1982). The national finding that two-thirds of CPNs were aged between 20 and 40 years and were the youngest of all nursing groups working in the community, reflected exactly the position of the six. Similarly, the national finding that 60 per cent of CPNs were male showed an exceptional preponderance of the gender and compared locally with half the study team. Eighty-one per cent of the national survey had worked as community psychiatric nurses for 5 years or less and compared with 83 per cent locally.

The recommended channel for making a non-urgent GP referral to an identified CPN was by letter. All referrals were understood to be for assessment in the first instance, followed by a CPN report to the GP advising on a course of action. Separate services existed for those under 16 years old, those over 75 years, and for the mentally handicapped, and were outside the interest of the present research.

Methods

Documents

Within the limits of the accuracy of available documents, the number of referrals from each of the 68 general practitioners to the six community psychiatric nurses received during the year ending 31 December 1981 was recorded and repeated both for the consultant psychiatrists and the nurse behavioural therapist (NBT). These data were related to general practitioner variables of practice size, list size, year of qualification and location of practice.

Semantic Differential

A fourteen scale semantic differential (Osgood *et al.*, 1957) was designed to measure the GP perceived characteristics of the service provided by community psychiatric nurses and six other occupational groups to whom GPs could refer psychologically distressed patients. It was posted to all GPs in the Health District and achieved a 72 per cent response by return, following one reminder letter. These data were related to general practitioner patterns of referral.

Interviews

Twenty-three GPs were interviewed to explore their attitude toward the management of those patients who present with psychological distress, the factors in play which influenced their decision to refer, and their choice of agency. A random stratified sample was drawn on the basis of their referral pattern to CPNs and to consultant psychiatrists provided by the documentary evidence, although conducted only with those prepared to be interviewed. Fourteen doctors declined and were, on average, some four years less experienced than those who agreed and the average for all sixty-eight GPs. However, the GPs who were interviewed were observed to share an identical rank order of agencies by semantic differential score as those who were not interviewed and, so too, the total number of semantic differential respondents. Interviews were conducted by the author who was guided by a schedule. Each was tape recorded, transcribed verbatim and subjected to content analysis.

Participant Observation

A 65-day period of participant observation was undertaken and reported elsewhere (White, 1983). Specific treatment and referral decisions were reported to, and patients interviewed by the on-site researcher (author). One hundred and eighty patients entered the study cohort by virtue of the GP's perception in surgery attenders, of a measure of psychological distress such that warranted further contact by them and/or referral to another agency. These data related the patients' personal characteristics and their psychological symptom patterns to general practitioner treatment decisions.

Computer programmes for the analysis of all data were written for the purpose by staff of the Statistical and Operational Research Department of a Regional Health Authority in England. Associations and differences between variables have not been quoted unless they reached statistical significance at the 5 per cent level or beyond, that is, unless the probability of an association or difference of such magnitude happening by chance was not more than 5 in 100. Standard Chi-square tests of association were used. The computer was an ICL 1904S.

Selected Findings

A total of 270 referrals were directly made to six community psychiatric nurses by sixty-eight general practitioners during one year. Each GP therefore referred on average four times, the range being between 0 and 18 (S.D. 3.8), and therefore each CPN received on average 45 referrals per annum. This compared with an average of almost twice that frequency of 7.75 occasions to consultant psychiatrists over the same period. For the nurse behavioural therapist, over three-quarters of the GPs in the District did not refer at all during the year and most of the remaining quarter did so only once. 41 per cent of the total number of referrals to the NBT came from one GP. Twice as many women were referred directly to the CPNs as men and, on average, were modestly older; males 41.7 years, females 45.5 years.

Strong evidence was revealed to show that GPs working in groups referred significantly more frequently to CPNs than those working alone or with a single partner. However, generalizations should not be made as there was only one 5-handed and one 6-handed general practice in the Health District. No evidence of differences was found for consultant psychiatrists.

No evidence was found to reveal significant differences in referral volume by the year in which the sixty-eight GPs qualified as doctors either for CPNs or consultant psychiatrists. However, GPs in urban practices were found to refer significantly more frequently, to both CPNs and consultant psychiatrists, than those in rural practices. More referrals were observed than were expected from GPs with midsized patient lists.

GPs guessed that about 20 per cent of surgery attenders experience primary psychological distress and claimed to hold largely counselling-like briefs involving listening, explaining, propping, and supporting. Two-fifths of the GPs considered available surgery time a limiting factor for both the quality and quantity of psychological work which was undertaken by them. However, independent of the time restriction believed to be related to relative list size, the overarching factor for some doctors remained individual interest and commitment to that aspect of general practice. While two-fifths of doctors were dissuaded from referral to any other agency if it were known there would be an unacceptable delay, 69 per cent of the sample claimed lack of time as the single most powerful factor present in treatment decisions which resulted in a referral outside general practice for psychologically distressed patients.

Three-fifths of GPs interviewed described negative, discouraging characteristics of the service provided by social workers to psychologically distressed patients referred to them. Over one-third used health visitors instead of, and in preference to, social workers. Half the GPs identified their perception of available CPN time as an inclining factor toward CPN referral and was widely regarded as a resource which could be marshalled to patients who were considered by GPs to be in need of it. Time was regarded, however, as a scarce resource of other agents, expressed particularly of those which were doctor-based, and referral to a CPN was often as an alternative to a time demand which might have otherwise been made on them. Similarly, almost half of the GPs were influenced to refer to a CPN by the relative speed with which the service could be delivered and was measured against what was seen as a lack of it in other agencies who might have been invited to provide a similar service.

The clear impression of the relative speed with which the CPNs mobilized the available time which they were believed to possess, was in sharp contrast to the understanding of the technical functions exercised during contact with patients referred to them, although more than two-thirds of the GPs found CPNs general assessment and counselling abilities attractive influencing factors. There was the view for 43 per cent, however, that the individual personal characteristics of the CPN were as, or more, important than qualification or title.

Three-quarters of GPs reported that contact with the CPN identified with their practices had been useful experience and nine-tenths of them reported that their own patient management or previous referral style had been affected by the opportunity to refer directly to a CPN. For three-quarters of them, it had meant that certain patients were being referred to a CPN who would have otherwise been referred to a consultant psychiatrist or dealt with by GPs themselves and who, on average, referred more frequently than those GPs who had not reported such experience.

Three-fifths of GPs first recalled a positive memorable experience of the service from a CPN and referred on average twice as many times as those that did not. Almost all the positive memorable experiences which were recalled first were related to a CPN treatment approach which had led to a referral outcome or direction which was perceived by the GP as successful and welcome, particularly when the perception was endorsed by the patient so referred. Occasionally, positive memorable experiences were of an unsuccessful referral outcome but were, nevertheless congruent with the GP's own previous treatment attempts and expectation of others. Almost three-fifths of the negative memorable experiences were reported of occasions when the clinical view or treatment style adopted by the CPN did not accord with that of the referring GP. Discrete evidence was found of a GP who had reported a negative memorable experience of the service from a CPN first, had claimed that contact had not been useful and work practice which had remained unaffected, although had referred two and a half times more frequently than the average for all the GPs in the Health District. Similarly, only 2.4 per cent of the variation in the number of referrals to CPNs could be explained by the variation in the semantic differential score for the service provided by a CPN. There were, therefore, large variations in GP referral behaviour which could not be explained by the CPN semantic differential scores.

Discussion

The health care of the community in the United Kingdom has been the responsibility of a number of occupational groups, although typically the pattern has been that an individual who experiences physical symptoms or anxieties will decide to visit the GP. The GP has then to decide whether to refer the individual to specialist services or deal with matters within the context of the primary health care team. The recent history of medicine as a series of struggles amongst group alliances and the historical dominance of the physicians, has meant that occupational groups which are more recently developed in the field of health care are forced to seek their mandate of operation not only from their clients and the State but also from the physician organizations. Furnham et al. (1981) has suggested that the distinction between those professions to whom physicians have devolved jurisdiction and those who were thought of as having appropriated it, have respectively characterized the historical experiences of nurses and social workers.

Unlike social workers and health visitors, nurses—including the community psychiatric nurses of the present study—have their access to patients controlled by a medical practitioner. Thus the medical profession has great influence over nurses' performance and development. Indeed, Dingwall (1974) dismissed nurses' claims to professional autonomy as a pipe dream on the grounds of that control in the community setting. Similarly, Bowling (1981) found GPs to be particularly reluctant to yield part of their role to non-physicians because of feelings of threat to independence and professionalism and fears of role encroachment. This, in spite of findings, mostly American and Canadian, which have revealed that nurse practitioners can safely and effectively, and with as much satisfaction to patients, provide first contact primary medical care (Marsh and Kaim Caudle, 1976; Linn, 1976; Nelson et al., 1974; Komaroff et al., 1974; Smith and Mottram, 1967; Smith and O'Donovan, 1970; Litman, 1972; Spitzer et al., 1974; Bailit et al., 1975). Opposition therefore to schemes which involved the use of non-physicians was understandable, Bowling argued, although illogical when so many doctors in general practice complained of lack of time.

Despite the possibility that available time was linked to patient list size, and that it was an aim of the British Medical Association (1982) to reduce lists to 1700, it was not known that smaller lists would necessarily lead GPs to devote more time to their patients, nor influence the effectiveness or humane quality of patient care (Merrison, 1979), nor necessarily become reflected in an improved rate of morbidity or mortality (Short, 1981). The present study observed CPN referral volume to be independent of any significant influence from GP list size.

The implicit assumption within a request for a CPN to devote time, in amounts either not available to the GP or to the patient, was that had such time—real or imaginary—been available, the GP would have dealt with matters. Therein rested the notion of delegation; that a request by a GP for a CPN to be in therapeutic contact with a patient on their list may contain the belief that the encounter is in lieu of contact with the doctor; simply, a delegate. Similarity may exist in the understanding of delegation and the notion of referral. Referral assumed that the referrer did not have the personal resource to deal with that which was presented and, further, had recognized that someone else may have; that is, even given infinite time, matters could not be appropriately dealt with without specific recourse to another. The meaning given to the notion of CPN referral may, therefore, sometimes contain elements more suited to the notion of delegation.

The interchangeable use of the two terms may explain how, on occasions, CPNs were tied by the expectation to be both therapeutically the same as GPs and therapeutically special and different. Examples were observed to show that some referrals which contained a prescriptive component, or a request for time, may have been considered by the GP as a request to undertake a delegated task. This may have run counter to the commonly known assessment brief held by all CPNs in the study and who could, therefore, revise or resist the conditions of the request— a contradiction of delegation—the result of which may have differed from the affirmation expected by the GP. Conversely, at times when the challenge of an alternative view was expected as a consequence of referral to a different agent, considered to be special, an endorsement of the existing view of the general practitioner may have served only to disappoint. In these circumstances which led to a struggle of expectations the GP held, and could therefore exercise, the means of influencing the development of the CPN potential.

In that sense, the GP became the customer of the CPN service and referral practice was influenced by both circumstances. A reduction in the referral volume as a consequence of either or both events was not uncommon. A less common effect was to continue to refer patients, occasionally in greater numbers than before, with whom nothing was thought therapeutically possible. The extension of both decisions was to reduce the opportunity open to CPNs to develop; on the one hand by limiting the access necessary for the recruitment of clients or on the other, by restricting referrals to those for whom there was thought no hope.

In order to stimulate referral from general practitioners, community psychiatric nurses were expected to demonstrate a wide brief and accept all-comers, much in the manner of the general practitioners themselves. Despite Merrison's (1979) view that GPs were free to select and reject a patient on their lists, this was not commonly endorsed. Indeed, the apparent privilege which occurred as a side-effect of the CPN assessment brief, to engage and discharge patients referred to them, was experienced by some GPs as a freedom not enjoyed by themselves. While the explanation may again lie in the disparate expectations which were implicit within the notions of delegation and referral, the pragmatic effect was to call for finer CPN role definition. As part of that process required attention to those aspects of the role which may have been considered outside that conceived by the CPN, either in terms of client group or the nature or period of contact, the definition risked a reduction in the wide, all-comers brief which GPs found attractive. The balance therefore, if not the paradox, was for CPNs to delineate their role satisfactorily and maintain the appeal of their service.

The substantial variations in the rate of referral from GPs to CPNs has shown mere volume to be an uncertain measure of the regard in which the service was held and suggested that the patterns may have been bereft of rationality. Examples were observed of the uniquely idiosyncratic nature of general practice which Barlow (1973) claimed was very much what the doctor decides to make it; that the field was enormous and that it all belonged to the GP who was literally answerable to nobody else. The present organization and management of general practitioner services has been through an independent contractual arrangement with Family Practitioner Committees (FPCs) which have survived despite a concerted lobby against their retention in response to the consultative document (DHSS, 1981b) which sought comment on the future arrangements for the administration of general practitioner services.

Strong opposition was recorded by the Royal College of Nursing of the United Kingdom (1981) and The Royal College of Midwives (1981) who expressed 'extreme disappointment' and 'regret' that the recommendation of the Royal Commission on the National Health Service (Merrison, 1979) to abolish FPCs and for their functions to be assumed by Health Authorities had been ignored. The Health Visitors Association (1981) was 'horrified' by the Governments decision. In all, sixty-eight commentators, including eight national bodies; two Regional Health Authorities; fifteen Area Health Authorities and thirty-two Community Health Councils (DHSS, 1981c) endorsed the recommendation of the Royal Commission. Nevertheless, the Conservative Government left unchanged the organizational arrangement for GPs and subjugated the objections raised by the organizations of the principal occupational groups involved with the provision of primary health care.

The case against FPCs, has been that their autonomous existence has prevented health care provision in an area being planned and administered as a whole (Rapoport, 1980). At present, Health Authorities plan for certain parts of health care provision—health visitors, district nurses, community psychiatric nurses—but cannot exercise any influence over the location or working arrangements of the medical practitioner who stands at the core of the primary health care team. As a result of this, GPs have retained a position of authority to continue to subordinate emergent health care groups to their own control and direction (Friedson, 1970; Johnson, 1972).

The caricature of CPNs was therefore of young men and women, specifically unqualified for, and reltively new to, the community setting, trading heavily on previous experiences gained in institutional environments with a lack of role definition based upon an independent body of knowledge. Thus, a broad similarity with GPs could be drawn. However, the inequality of the power and prestige positions of both groups remained to offset otherwise common denominations. Referral volume, from one to the other, reflected one imperfect measure of the individual manner in which both the personal and role characteristics of the CPN had been originally presented, reviewed in the light of subsequent experience and variously accommodated by GPs. The relative extent to which the accommodation took place was influenced by the nature of the contact behaviour between both agencies. Contact provided the forum for the pairs of individuals to become personally and professionally acquainted and, thereafter, influenced the manner in which referral outcome was eventually perceived by GPs. An endorsement of the CPN service from the patients so referred, drawn from those who would have otherwise been treated by GP's themselves or, not uncommonly, by consultant psychiatrists, was an important element in the validation of general practitioner decisions to request CPN intervention. A close proximity to GPs was generally welcomed and it was shown that the dividend for CPNs in so doing stimulated an increase in referral volume. The converse may also partly explain the pattern of GPs who were dormant or infrequent referrers both to CPNs and especially to the nurse behaviour therapist.

A demonstration of flexibility which resulted from useful contact, and the preparedness of CPN's to accept task-orientated requests, enhanced the likelihood of multiple referral. As a consequence, however, discrete evidence of intrinsic and extrinsic role overlap was apparent both for CPNs and other nursing-based groups, particularly with social work. Explanation for this may be anchored in the short history of community psychiatric nursing given that part of their original raison d'être was in response to missing social work functions. However, where the nature of the role ambiguity resulted from expedient imputation, CPN's, while seeking an independent position in the 'medical' division of labour, may not avoid a workload, as Dingwall (1974) suggested, of a heterogeneous collection of tasks discarded by physicians—a diluted medicine. The strong reference to limited GP time as a powerful influencing factor for referral to CPNs may, therefore, contain early elements of Dingwall's observation.

The acknowledgement of GPs' lack of homogeneity was further reflected in the present study in the wide variation of individual interest in psychiatry and uses made of services connected with it. However, the present organizational arrangement of GPs, and community psychiatric nurses in relation to them, has provided a scenario which may result in the CPN role and function being substantially and variously influenced by doctor definition outside hospitals as it has been, historically, inside them. The size, range and nature of referrals to CPNs may not, therefore, mirror so much the characteristics of the catchment population, as the title may imply, but rather the heterogeneous characteristics of the referring GPs. The limits to the potential contribution to the health care of the community may not, therefore, have been eventually restricted by skill, but by the relative resourcefulness of individual nurse practitioners to negotiate cooperative terms with GPs which would allow access to suitable consumers.

Summary

Historically, community psychiatric nurses in the United Kingdom have been based in psychiatric hospitals and offered services to patients referred to them principally by consultant psychiatrists. More recently, there has been a movement toward their closer involvement with primary care givers and to the acceptance of direct referrals from general practitioners. Little was known about what influenced the work demands made upon community psychiatric nurses by general practitioners, and more information was thus required.

Four research methods were designed and employed to focus on the referral practices of, and the relationships between, general practitioners and community psychiatric nurses. Information was gathered from documents which recorded the volume of CPN referral, during one year, from all 68 GPs who practiced in one south coast District Health Authority in England. This was complemented by information provided from a postal semantic differential returned by three-quarters of the GP population. Interviews were also conducted with a third of all GPs, together with a period of participant observation with a tenth.

The findings have shown that the spread of attitudes toward psychologically distressed surgery attenders and the range of strategies for dealing with them reflected the individual and independent nature of general practice. Wide variation in direct referral rates to community psychiatric nurses were observed in patterns independent of most variables except the nature of individually negotiated working relationships. Each was influenced by the nature of the contact behaviour between both groups and by the congruence between the expectation and experience of referral outcomes. In circumstances which led to a struggle of expectations, the present disparate organizational arrangements and the power relations between doctors and nurses meant that GPs held, and could therefore exercise, the means of influencing the development of the CPN role potential. The quality and quantity of referrals to CPNs was thus found to be a function of their specific relationship with GPs.

References

Bailit, H., Lewis, J., Hochneiser, L., and Bush, N. (1975) Assessing the quality of care. *Nursing Outlook*, **23**, 153–159.

Barker, C. (1981). Into the community. *Health and Social Service Journal*, **20**, 315–318.

Barlow, D. T. C. (1973). *British General Practice*. H. K. Lewis, London.

Bowling, A. (1981). *Delegation in General Practice*. Tavistock Publications, London.

Brearley, P., Gibbons, J., Miles, A., Topliss, E., and Woods, G. (1978). *The Social Context of Health Care*. Basil Blackwell, Oxford.

British Medical Association (1982). Family Practitioner Committees under scrutiny (press release). *Health and Social Service Journal*, **92**, 872.

Brook, P., and Cooper, B., (1975). Community mental health: primary team and specialist services. *Journal of the Royal College of General Practitioners*, **25**, 93–110.

Cartwright, A. and Anderson, R. (1981). *General Practice Revisited*. Tavistock Publications, London.

Clyne, M. B. (1974). How personal is the personal care in General Practice? (Quoted from Professor Walton, Department of Psychiatry, University of Edinburgh.) *Journal of Royal College of General Practitioners*, **24**, 263–266.

Community Psychiatric Nurses Association (1981). *Community Psychiatric Nursing Services Survey*. (Often read with a companion document 'Directory'). Community Psychiatric Nurses Association.

Corser, C. M. and Ryce, S. W., (1977). Community mental health care: a model based on the primary care system. *British Medical Journal*, **2**, 936–938.

Department of Health and Social Security (1975). *Better Services for the Mentally Ill*. HMSO, London.

Department of Health and Social Security (1976). *Priorities for Health and Personal Social Services in England: A consultative document*. HMSO, London.

Department of Health and Social Security (1981a). *Care in the community. A Consultative Document on Moving Resources for Care in England*. July. DHSS, London.

Department of Health and Social Security (1981b). Health Notice HN(81)10. *Arrangements for the Administration of Family Practitioner Services: A consultative paper*. DHSS, London.

Department of Health and Social Security (1981c). *Arrangements for the Administration of Family Practitioner services*. Summary of comments on consultative paper HN(81)10. RL1A GCD139/J11. DHSS, London.

Dingwall, R. (1974). Some sociological aspects of nursing research. *Sociological Review*, 22, 1.

Drury, M. and Hull, R. (1979). *Introduction to General Practice*. Bailliere Tindall, London.

Dunnell, K. and Dobbs, J. (1982). Nurses working in the community. Office of Populations, Census and Surveys. HMSO, London.

Friedson, F. (1970). *Profession of Medicine*. Dodd, New York.

Furnham, A., Pendleton, D., and Manican, C. (1981). The perception of different occupations within the medical profession. *Social Science and Medicine*, **15**, 289–300.

Goldberg, D. (1982). Personal correspondence.

Goldberg, D. and Blackwell, B. (1970). Psychiatric illness in general practice. A detailed study using a new method of case identification. *British Medical Journal*, **2**, 439–43.

Goldberg, D. and Huxley, P. (1980). *Mental Illness in the Community: the Pathway to Psychiatric Care*. Tavistock Publications, London.

Greene, J. (1968). The psychiatric nurse in the community. *International Journal of Nursing Studies*, **5**, 175–183.

Griffith, J. H. and Mangen, S. P. (1980). Community psychiatric nursing — a literature review. *International Journal of Nursing Studies*, **17**, 197–210.

Harker, P., Leopoldt, H., and Robinson, J. R. (1976). Attaching community psychiatric nurses to general practice. *Journal of the Royal College of General Practitioners*, **26**, 170.

Health Visitors Association (1981). *Comments on the Consultative Paper on Arrangements for the Administration of Family Practitioner Services.* HN(81)10, JKW/JKC, May. HVA, London.

Hunter, P. (1959). The changing function of professional staff in the mental hospital, in *Ventures of Professional Co-operation.* Association of Professional Social Workers, London.

Hunter, P. (1978). *Schizophrenia and Community Psychiatric Nursing.* National Schizophrenia Fellowship.

Johnson D. (1973). Treatment of depression in general practice. *British Medical Journal,* **2,** 18-20.

Johnson, D. (1974). A study of the use of antidepressant medication in general practice. *British Journal of Psychiatry,* **125,** 186-192.

Johnson, T. (1972). *Professions and Power.* Macmillan, London.

Jones, K., Brown, J. and Bradshaw J., (1978). *Issues in Social Policy.* Routledge and Kegan Paul, London.

Kaeser, A. C. and Cooper, B., (1971). The psychiatric patient, the general practitioner and the outpatient clinic: an operational study and review. *Psychological Medicine,* **1,** 312-325.

Kessel, W. I. N. (1960). Psychiatric morbidity in a London general practice. *British Journal of Preventive and Social Medicine,* **14,** 16-22.

Komaroff, A. L., Black, W. L., Flatley, M., Knopp, R. H., Reiffen, B., and Sherman, H. (1974). Protocols for Physicians Assistants. *New England Journal of Medicine,* **290,** 307-312.

Linn, L. S. (1976). Patient acceptance of the Family Nurse Practitioner. *Medical Care,* **14,** 357-364.

Litman, T. J. (1972). Public perceptions of the Physicians Assistant. *American Journal of Public Health,* **62,** 343-346.

Marsh, G. N. and Kaim Caudle, P. (1976). *Team Care in General Practice.* Croom Helm, London.

May, A. R. (1965). The psychiatric nurse in the community. *Nursing Mirror,* 31 December, 409-410.

May, A. R. and Gregory, E. (1968). Participation of General Practitioners in community psychiatry. *British Medical Journal,* 168-171.

May, A. R. and Moore, S. (1963). The mental nurse in the community. *The Lancet,* 26 January, 213-214.

Merrison, A. (1979). *Report on the Royal Commission on the National Health Service.* HMSO, London.

Moore, S. (1961). A psychiatric out-patient nursing service. *Mental Health Bulletin,* Summer.

Nelson, E. C., Jacobs, A. R., and Johnson, K. G. (1974). Patients' acceptance of Physicians Assistants. *Journal of the American Medical Association,* **228,** 63-67.

Osgood, C. E., Suci, G. J. and Tannenbaum, P. H. (1957). *The measurement of Meaning.* University of Illinois Press, Urbana.

Pilkington, H. (1960). *Report of the Royal Commission on Doctors and Dentists Remuneration,* Cmnd. 939. HMSO, London.

Powell, E. (1961). In *Emerging Patterns for the Mental Health Services and the Public.* Proceedings of a conference, 9-10 March. National Association for Mental Health, London.

232 PSYCHIATRIC NURSING RESEARCH

Rapoport, M. (1980). A salaried GP service in the cities. *Medicine in Society*, Autumn/Winter, 10-11, London.

Rawnsley, K. and Loundon, J. (1962). The attitudes of general practitioners to psychiatry, in P. Halmos (Ed.), *Sociology and Medicine, Sociological Review*, Monograph No. 5. University of Keele.

Reynolds, R. E. and Bice, T. W. (1971). Attitudes of Medical Interns towards patients and health professionals. *Journal of Health and Social Behaviour*, **12** 307-311.

Robertson, N. (1979). Variations in referral pattern to the psychiatric services by general practitioners. *Psychological Medicine*, **9**, 355-364.

Royal College of General Practitioners (1981). *Prevention of Psychiatric Disorders in General Practice*. Report from general practice 20. Royal College of General Practitioners, London.

Royal College of Midwives (1981). Comments on Health Services Development HN(81)10: Arrangements for the administration of Family Practitioner Services. A consultative paper. RCM/209/81, June. RCM, London.

Royal College of Nursing of the United Kingdom, (1981). Comments on the DHSS consultative paper on the arrangements for the administration of Family Practitioner Services, DHR/MH/PHCS, May. RCN, London.

Sencicle, L. (1981). Which way the CPN? *Community Psychiatric Nurses Association Journal*, January/February, 10-14.

Shaw, A. (1975). CPN attachment to group practice. *Nursing Times*, **73** (12). Health Centre Supplement 9-14.

Shepherd, M., Cooper, B., Brown, A. C. and Kalton, G. W. (1966). *Psychiatric Illness in General Practice*. Oxford University Press, London.

Short, R. (1981). *Fourth Report from the Social Services Committee: Medical Education*. HMSO, London.

Smith, J. W. and Mottram, E. M. (1967). Extending use of nursing services in general practice. *British Medical Journal*, **4**, 672-674.

Smith, J. W. and O'Donovan, J. B. (1970). The Practice Nurse — A new look. *British Medical Journal*, **IV**, 673-677.

Spitzer, W. O., Sackett, D. L., Sibley, J. C., Roberts, R. S., Gent, M., Kergin, D. J., Hackett, B. C. and Olynich, A. (1974). The Burlington Randomised Trial of the Nurse Practitioner. *New England Journal of Medicine*, **290**, 251-256.

Titmuss, R. (1961). Community care — fact or fiction?, in *Emerging Patterns for the Mental Health Services and the Public*. Report of the annual conference of the National Association for Mental Health. MIND, London.

Walton, H. J. (1966). Differences between physically-minded and psychologically-minded medical practitioners. *British Journal of Psychiatry*, **112**, 1097-1102.

Walton, H. J. (1969). Effects of the doctors personality on his style of practice. *Journal of the Royal College of General Practitioners*, **82**, Suppl. 3, 6-17.

Warren, J. (1971). Long acting phenothiazine injections given by psychiatric nurses in the community. *Nursing Times*, **67**, Occasional Paper, 141-143.

White, E. G. (1983). 'If its beyond me . . .': community psychiatric nurses in relation to general practice. MSc Thesis (Social Policy). Cranfield Institute, England.

Williams, P. (1979). *The Interface Between Psychiatry and General Practice*. S.K.F. publications, vol. 2, No. 7.

CHAPTER 13

The Effectiveness of Community Psychiatric Nursing Teams and Base-locations

DAVID SKIDMORE

Editor's Comments

David Skidmore used observation, interviews, and analysis of re-cords to examine the relationship between CPN base-locations and methods of practice. He studied hospital-based CPN teams and primary health care-based CPN teams, but found no differences in intervention styles.

The chapter highlights many issues important for the development of community psychiatric nursing. For example, David Skidmore describes how the nurses were obviously ill-prepared for their role, resorting to institutional and coercive methods of care. He argues that CPNs need more specialized training, particularly skills training.

Introduction

It has been suggested that Community Psychiatric Nursing (CPN) in the United Kingdom commenced at Warlingham Park Hospital in 1954 (Sharpe, 1982). However, the rapid expansion of this service appears to have had its genesis some ten years later because of various political and economic influences:

1   Government legislation during the 1960s which attempted to effect changes in the health services helped to formalize the concept of community care (DHSS, 1962).

233

2 The introduction of long-acting phenothiazine drugs during the 1960s.

3 The implications of the Seebohm Report (1972) appeared to leave a void in the area of mental health.

By 1966 a total of 46 psychiatric hospitals were using staff in community care, rising to 163 by 1980 (Community Psychiatric Nurses' Association (CPNA), 1981). Friend (1985) argues that the expansion of the CPN service led to a diversity of bases without apparent direction. Some schools of thought boldly insisted that Primary Health Care Teams (PHCT) were ideal bases (Leopoldt, 1975; Shaw, 1977), while others doggedly retained hospital anchorage. Concomitant with this is the notion that CPNs are inadequately trained for their role (Skidmore and Friend, 1984). Sharpe (1982) suggests that there is a national trend towards the PHCT and implicit preventative care, although a national survey conducted by the CPNA (1982) revealed that 75 per cent of teams were still hospital based; 8 per cent PHCT based and 17 per cent had dual bases. The same survey revealed that 54 per cent of respondants felt that a dual base was the ideal location, 29 per cent the PHCT, 4 per cent the hospital, and 13 per cent were unsure.

The ideal location for CPNs, in terms of needs and effectiveness, has, apparently, never been evaluated. Consequently the CPN service is still developing in juxtaposition. The majority of CPN teams are hospital based. These nurses are employed by the psychiatric institution and may fail to gain experience of other community agencies. They are 'protected' by the 'mother' hospital in that they have all the resources of that hospital to fall back on. It could be argued that many of these nurses are not versed in the skills deemed necessary for successful intervention in the community (Butterworth and Skidmore, 1981; Skidmore and Friend, 1984). It has been suggested that such nurses may view the community as an extension of the institution (Golan, 1978). One could argue that starved of the philosophies of veteran community workers they only have their own experience of institutional care to build upon. Coupled with this is the notion that hospital teams rarely have the opportunity for preventative work, if referrals are controlled by consultant psychiatrists. It has been argued that hospital care bears no relation to community care (Butterworth and Skidmore, 1981).

Conversely, a CPN service which has developed in the community and is attached to a PHCT tends to be somewhat isolated from a large 'mother hospital' and, by necessity, would be required to develop its own resources. Such a team would have ready access to the veteran community worker and have ample opportunity to observe methods and be exposed to philosophies that did not arise from institutions. Carr *et al.* (1980) argue that the education of CPNs should be exposing them to models of care other than the medical model, which has been a formative influence on nursing roles. One could also argue that the PHCT is an ideal base for preventative intervention.

Skidmore (1980) suggests that 75 per cent of self-referrals to a GP clinic are of a non-medical nature; often for advice regarding a personal problem. The GP lacks the time and training to cope effectively with these and either refers to a psychiatrist or prescribes drugs (Doyle, 1982). A logical step would be to refer such patients to the CPN service. Skidmore (1980) also suggests that 'clients' of the health caring professions indicate a preference and feel more satisfied with community centred care rather than with institutional care; this feeling appears to be projected onto the agents of either arena.

It can be argued that the approach and attitude to care delivery adopted by the professional is paramount when attempting to motivate a positive attitude in clients. There is a surfeit of evidence which suggests that institutions and their professionals fail in their attempts to produce client-satisfaction and lack of anxiety (Cassell, 1978; Miller, 1978; Bradshaw, 1978). Stimson and Webb (1975) argue that the approach a client takes to a medical encounter determines satisfaction regarding the outcome of such an encounter. One could further suggest that this is equally true of the stance taken by the professional. Skidmore (1980) indicated a clear dichotomy in the way that both clients and professionals approached institutional and community-based encounters. The approach to the institution led to a largely negative outcome and was reflected in clients' accounts of their satisfaction; the approach towards the community was quite the reverse. If the 'negative-institutional' response can be transferred into the community, as Golan (1978) suggests, then one would expect to observe differences in intervention techniques between the two philosophies.

The institution demands passivity from its clients (Goffman, 1963; Illich, 1974; Bradshaw, 1978; Butterworth and Skidmore, 1981) and it is suggested that sanctions are applied if a client does not conform to the passive role (Stockwell, 1972). However, the community-based therapeutic regime demands a more active role of the client since the twenty-four hour cover offered in the institution is not available. Clients, by necessity, are required to take more responsibility for their own treatment (Skidmore and Stoker, 1974). Arguably, such differences may be identified by comparing methods of intervention, reasons of referral, and case-load management.

The Study

The uncertainty of location coupled with the cry for mandatory training prompted the institution of this study in 1980. The principal aims were to evaluate and identify any differences between the styles of interventions and philosophies within the two types of CPN bases; and to examine the notion that PHCT bases prompted more intervention of a preventative nature.

The Sample

For the purpose of this study three types of bases were identified:

1   A CPN team which was totally hospital based, consultant attached, and managed by a hospital nursing officer.
2   A totally PHCT-based service, operating an open-referral system.
3   A team which had a dual base and had a two-way referral system (consultants and GPs).

A total of twelve teams were identified; from this sample it was possible to match six teams with regard to sex-ratio, age, experience, and qualifications. Consequently, six teams, two from each area described above, were studied in depth for a thirty-month period. The sample consisted of sixty CPNs: thirty were hospital based; sixteen dual based and fourteen PHCT based.

The Methods

The methods used in this study were:

1   Non-participant observation so that the CPN's style of approach could be witnessed and contact time determined.
2   Content analysis of referrals, to determine the reasons for referral and outcome.
3   Open interview, to determine the philosophy of operational style and attitudes towards intervention techniques.

The Results

Approximately one thousand hours of observations were recorded within the various teams and five thousand referrals were analysed. All team members cooperated fully with members of the research team.

Primarily, it should be stated that the expectations of differences in practice between teams were not realized. No significant differences were found in intervention strategies between teams. All teams boasted similar styles of intervention: group therapy, behavioural therapy, and family therapy; however, these particular intervention styles were normally prompted by individual team members rather than being the inherent philosophy of the various teams.

No significant differences were found between teams concerning reasons for visits; the main reasons proffered were assessment, support, and treatment. Other reasons were identified by the observations such as delivering medication, messages and student teaching, and these occurred in all teams.

Similarly, there existed no marked differences between the size and content of case-loads. The average case-load of all team members was forty and 70 per cent of the intervention was of a 'supportive' nature in all teams. The reasons for referrals also displayed no marked differences between teams. The majority of cases (90 per cent of 5000) had previous psychiatric involvement and were referred to by the practitioners as 'old' cases. Only 10 per cent of all referrals were termed 'new' in that they had no previous psychiatric involvement, and of these 60 per cent were re-referred to other agencies (social workers and marriage guidance). Consequently, the notion of preventative involvement was also negated. Although 100 per cent of this sample, on interview, maintained that families were always involved, when possible, only 30 per cent of families within the referral sample analysed were contacted and these were equally distributed throughout the teams and not influenced by CPN base-location.

On interview, 68 per cent of the CPNs stated that they were not sufficiently prepared or educated to take on the changing style of psychiatric referrals (these were seen to be increasingly of a personal/ relationship problem). Consequently, the CPNs maintained their contact in the 'safe' area of tertiary care; 75 per cent of this sample maintained that they lacked the necessary skills to develop preventative work.

The CPNs with PHCT commitment admitted that GPs had tried to involve them in counselling clients prior to psychiatric referral, but the CPNs had referred such clients to other agencies because of their own inadequacies. Eventually the GPs stopped referring this type of client and reverted to 'supportive' referrals and injection referrals. Interestingly, all CPNs interviewed experienced difficulty in defining what they meant by 'support'. Responses ranged from 'surveillance' to 'checking for side-effects from drugs'.

Discussion

Although the base-location appears to be irrelevant regarding the effectiveness of CPN teams, one would argue that other areas highlighted by this study are worthy of further consideration. Primarily, one should consider that all CPNs, regardless of base, are derived from one common pool—the RMN syllabus. Of this sample, not one nurse had received any instruction/training in preparation for the community role and consequently had to rely on skills developed within the previous institutional role. In this respect Golan (1978) would be right in suggesting that the institution is being transferred into the community. By their own admission, CPNs lacked the skills to cope with clients who differed from those of which they had had previous experiences. The level of case involvement supported this notion and on interview 80 per cent of the CPNs admitted that they felt more 'comfortable' with established clients. The practising CPNs, of this sample, did not have the benefit of the new RMN syllabus, which may have prepared them, to some degree, for a community role. Consequently, all their experience was 'locked' in institutional care. Arguably, this may be why families were not normally involved in care programmes since it is not normal practice within institutional care. Eighty per cent of CPNs stated that families were not available during the hours of their visits. In fact 60 per cent of visits, observed, involved a family member going into another room in order to 'leave the professional to it'.

It might be argued that the advent of the Joint Board of Clinical Nursing Studies (JBCNS), now the English National Board (ENB) course 810 (Psychiatric Nursing in the Community), would have some influence on intervention. However, 30 per cent of this sample had undertaken such a course and no significant differences were noted between this group and their community counterparts who had not completed such a course.

Client-contact

One of the more alarming observations concerned client/CPN interaction. Although CPNs verbally supported the notions of non-directive counselling and self-responsibility for clients, little evidence for this could be found. Indeed, in several instances quite the reverse was noted and clients who questioned or disagreed were sanctioned by the threat of isolation:

'If you're not prepared to cooperate, there's no point in me coming to see you!'
'There's no need for me to keep coming if you've got it all worked out yourself.'

Even more disturbing, the CPNs appeared to be unaware of doing this and would leave such an encounter reiterating:

'Did you see how I let them make their own decision . . . you have to encourage them to take responsibility for themselves.'

Similarly, when clients on long-acting phenothiazines questioned or refused their medication, they were not encouraged to discuss their reasons but coerced by veiled threats:

'If you stop taking this you'll have to go back to hospital.'
'I'll have to tell the doctor!'
'It doesn't matter how long you have to take it as long as it keeps you out of hospital.'
'If you're going to be difficult about it you'll have to go up to the hospital to have it!'

There was also evidence of CPNs collaborating with relatives to control clients. Relatives tended to report 'difficulties' to CPNs in secret and their reports were usually accepted without question. Consequently, one was inclined to see the CPN as an agent of social control, marshalling the client into prescribed patterns of behaviour defined by relatives.

Another aspect of client-contact which caused concern was the amount of time spent with 'old' clients as opposed to 'new' clients. The average time spent with new clients, normally for the purposes of assessment, was fourteen minutes, as opposed to thirty-six minutes with old clients. On interview, much of the client assessment appeared to be carried out by sterotyping or intuitively:

' . . . you get a feeling . . . '
'You know they're depressed . . . '
'I've got a fairly clear picture from the relatives . . . '
'You can tell . . . as soon as you meet them.'

Conversely, the amount of time spent with old clients tended to be filled with everyday conversation, such sessions tending to be very friendly and informal, although no real material aid appeared to be offered.

'Well, I just call in now and again to make sure things are okay.'
'I drop by just in case any problems arise.'

Finally, the most informative part of the data related to the CPNs own misgivings concerning their roles. Seventy per cent of this sample maintained that they were inadequately trained for their 'community' role, even after they had completed the ENB 810 course.

'The course gets you thinking in a certain way, but doesn't tell
you what to do with these thoughts.'
'I feel out of my depth most of the time.'
'What we need are the skills to do the job . . . you're never
shown.'

It has been previously stated that all teams in this study boasted 'specialist'
skills, however, misgivings about such skills transpired:

'It's all I can offer and I get successes . . . but I get clients who
don't meet the criteria for groups . . . I don't really know what
to do with them!'
'I find that most people I start on behavioural programmes
don't really need it!'

To summarize the findings, then, this study illustrated that CPNs lacked
the skills to effectively carry out their roles; they often resorted to
institutional methods of care; an element of social control was evident;
the base-location had no significance regarding practice and methods used,
and training (ENB 810) had no significant influence on practice.

Conclusions

Primarily, it should be emphasized that these findings apply only to six
CPN teams in a specific area of the country; consequently, it should not
be assumed that all teams are alike. However, from this study one could
suggest that the education of the CPN requires a radical rethink.
Historically, CPNs have inherited a training that others think they require;
training has not, to date, been based on any evaluation of needs. In this
particular study the need for skills-training was certainly highlighted, and
this is one aspect of training that is markedly absent for CPNs. The ENB
810 course is largely an academic course that only glimpses at the various
skills required for effective practice.

One could argue that the CPN would ideally be placed within the PHCT
with respect to first time referrals. Not only would this reduce the risk
of clients 'getting lost' in the psychiatric system, but it could also reduce
the demand upon GPs' time. That there is a need for some kind of
intervention in this area is suggested by the amount of psychotropic drugs
prescribed in this arena (Parrish, 1972). The GP lacks the time to do
anything other than prescribe or refer. Evidence suggests that a large
percentage of self-referrals to GPs are for non-medical reasons (Skidmore,

1980) and it has been argued that many psychiatric problems are secondary to life-crises (Szasz, 1972; Larder, 1977; Cassell, 1978). One could suggest that such problems can be dealt with by effective counselling and thus reduce the demand on GP time and pharmaceutical bills. The CPN attached to the PHCT could be such a counsellor with the appropriate training. At present, the system appears to offer no alternative, CPNs are not trained to deal with these problems. One would argue that the PHCT could be the ideal base for the appropriately trained CPN. Primarily, they would be situated on the doorstep of the community, which could encourage self-referral. The stigma, still associated with psychiatric hospitals, would not necessarily contaminate them. They would also be well situated in order to plan strategies for more preventative work, i.e. health education and self-referral. However, such bases would prove irrelevant under the present system while CPNs are nowhere near meeting the needs of the community. By their own admission, and by analysis of case-loads, it can be deduced that they are not developing in a practical sense. Keeping the patient in the community is in vogue for both practical and economic reasons. The motivation to close the large mental hospitals (rightly or wrongly) is with us and will undoubtedly be realized. At present there appears to be little to replace it. While it has to be accepted that psychiatric hospitals caused much damage in terms of institutionalization and the image of psychiatric dysfunction, it must also be accepted that they created a need in society. While it is commendable that society is motivated to terminate their existence the needs of those who require constructive support, guidance, and rehabilitation should be considered. Is a conundrum to be replaced by a void? If this study is representative of the national trend, there can be no doubt. CPNs can only cope effectively with the 'professional' client, i.e. those with previous experience of psychiatry. If this resource is removed then the CPN could be totally redundant a few years later. This would in itself be a tragedy, since there is a specific role for them to play.

In the tradition of non-directive counselling one would recommend that CPNs set their own house in order. They are aware of their own shortcomings, only they can become aware of the needs of the community they serve. If training for CPNs is to be effective it must be based on needs. Consequently, there is an urgent demand for further research which identifies the needs of the community and its agents. Such findings can then be fed into an adequate skills-based course. One might then witness a change in the effectiveness of CPN teams.

This study suggests that skills are needed before CPNs can effectively carry out their role; it further implies that the existing system of training, both experientially and academic, falls short in meeting the needs of practitioners. Consequently, one cannot support the call for mandatory training and further expansion unless the system visibly changes. The system can only change via further study. The CPNs of this study had the courage to admit that they were deficient in their role; this admission probably requires more courage than it takes to do something about it. They are on the front line of training for the community hence they have a significant contribution to make.

Summary

In an attempt to identify the effectiveness of community psychiatric nursing base-locations, three community psychiatric nursing teams, from diverse bases, were matched with regard to qualification, sex, and case-loads. The teams were studied in depth over a period of thirty months; their methods of practice was observed, practitioners were interviewed, case-loads and referrals were analysed. The original brief of the study was to identify differences between hospital and primary health care bases; there was an assumption that such a difference would exist due to differing philosophies of practice. However, no significant differences were identified between methods of practice and base-location but the study did highlight several issues which are considered to be of great importance for the future education and further development of community psychiatric nurses. The results of this study suggest that all community psychiatric nurses require a more 'skills-based' education if they are to practice effectively and that the existing methods of training/ education fall short in preparing the nurse to meet the needs of clients in the community.

References

Bradshaw, J. (1978). *Doctors on Trial*. Wildwood, London.
Butterworth, C. A. and Skidmore, D. (1981). *Caring for the Mentally Ill in the Community*. Croom Helm, London.
Carr, P. J., Butterworth, C. A. and Hodges, B. E. (1980). *Community Psychiatric Nursing*. Churchill Livingstone, London.
Cassell, E. J. (1978).*The Healer's Art*. Pelican, Penguin Books, Harmondsworth, Middlesex.
Community Psychiatric Nurses Association (1981). *Report No. 8008*. CPNA, Leeds.
Community Psychiatric Nurses Association (1982). *Mandatory Training Survey*, Unpublished Survey. CPNA/Manchester Polytechnic.
D.H.S.S. (1962). *The Way Forward*, HMSO, London.

Doyle, C. (1982). *Prescribing Habits of GPs*. Research proposal for M. Phil, Manchester Polytechnic.

Friend, W. (1985). *CPN Effectiveness*. M. Phil Thesis, forthcoming, Manchester Polytechnic.

Goffman, I. (1963). *Stigma*. Pelican, Penguin Books, Harmondsworth, Middlesex.

Golan, N. (1978). *Treatment in Crisis Situations*. Macmillan, London.

Illich, I. (1974). *The Limits to Medicine*. Pelican, Penguin Books, Harmondsworth, Middlesex.

Larder, M. (1977). *Psychiatry on Trial*. Pelican, Penguin Books, Harmondsworth, Middlesex.

Leopoldt, H. (1975). Attachment and psychiatric domiciliary attachment. *Nursing Mirror*, **141**, 82–84.

Miller, J. (1978). *The Body in Question*. Cape, London.

Parrish, P. A. (1972). Prescribing of psychotropic drugs in General Practice. *Journal of the Royal College of General Practitioners*, suppl. 4, 92.

Seebohm Report (1972). *Committee on Local Authority and Allied Personal Social Series*. Cmnd 3703. HMSO, London.

Sharpe, D. (1982). GPs views of community psychiatric nurses. *Nursing Times*, **78**, 1664–1666.

Shaw, A. (1977). CPN attachment in group practice. *Nursing Times Health Care Supplement*, **73**, 12.

Skidmore, D. (1980). *The Hidden Machine*. Verus Microfiche.

Skidmore, D. and Friend, W. (1984). Muddling through. *Community Outlook*, 9 May, 179–181.

Skidmore, D. and Stoker, M. J. (1974). Space age therapy. *New Psychiatry*, **1** (4), 15–16.

Stimson, G. and Webb, B. (1975). *Going to See the Doctor*. Routledge and Kegan Paul, London.

Stockwell, F. (1972). *The Unpopular Patient*. Royal College of Nursing, Research Monograph, London.

Szasz, T. (1972). *The Myth of Mental Illness*. Granada, Herts.

Index